Revision Notes for the Resp
Specialty Certificate Exam~~ination~~

Revision Notes for the Respiratory Medicine Specialty Certificate Examination

Dr Caroline Patterson MRCP

Specialty Trainee in Respiratory Medicine; North West Thames Rotation

Dr Meg Coleman MRCP

Specialty Trainee in Respiratory Medicine; North West Thames Rotation

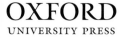

OXFORD

UNIVERSITY PRESS

Great Clarendon Street, Oxford, OX2 6DP,
United Kingdom

Oxford University Press is a department of the University of Oxford.
It furthers the University's objective of excellence in research, scholarship,
and education by publishing worldwide. Oxford is a registered trade mark of
Oxford University Press in the UK and in certain other countries

© Oxford University Press 2012

The moral rights of the authors have been asserted

First Edition published in 2012

Impression: 1

British Library Cataloguing in Publication Data

Data available

Library of Congress Cataloging in Publication Data

Library of Congress Control Number: 2012938467

ISBN 978-0-19-969348-1

Printed and bound by
CPI Group (UK) Ltd, Croydon, CR0 4YY

PREFACE

The Royal College of Physicians (RCP) introduced the Specialty Certificate Examination (SCE) in Respiratory Medicine in 2008. Passing this examination is mandatory for completion of specialty training and progression to becoming a Consultant.

This book is intended as a revision aid for candidates preparing for the Respiratory Medicine SCE. The authors were amongst the second cohort of candidates to sit the examination and have drawn upon their experience to assist others in achieving a successful outcome. Furthermore, it is anticipated that the book will be useful to anyone wishing to gain an overview of Respiratory Medicine.

The book uses the Specialty Training Curriculum for Respiratory Medicine, published by the Joint Royal Colleges of Physicians Training Board (JRCPTB), as the basis for a précis of current guidelines and practice in respiratory medicine. Relevant guidelines are highlighted throughout the text. Questions similar to those featured in the SCE are provided with answers and explanatory notes.

The SCE is a computer-based test, comprising two 3-hour papers, each with a total of 100 questions. The questions are of the 'best of five' multiple choice format. The RCP have suggested the questions will be distributed across the curriculum as follows:

Table 1

Topic	Number of questions (total 200)
Asthma	5
Chronic obstructive pulmonary disease	20
Thoracic oncology	20
Pulmonary infections	20
Tuberculosis and opportunistic mycobacterial disease	10
Cystic fibrosis	5
Diffuse parenchymal lung disease (interstitial lung disease)	25
Pulmonary vascular disease	15
Sleep-related breathing disorders and hypoventilation	5
Disorders of the pleura and mediastinum	15
Occupational and environmental lung disease	10
Physiology	20
Imaging	20
Other	10

This book should not be considered an exhaustive text but is intended to provide candidates with knowledge that is reasonably needed to pass the SCE, plus suggested references for further reading. Candidates' chances of success will be enhanced by clinical experience and engagement with the multidisciplinary team.

The authors are grateful to their own multidisciplinary teams for assistance in completing this book. Specific acknowledgement goes to Drs Gillian Bain and Olga Lazoura for their radiological images.

Good luck!
CP & MC

CONTENTS

6MWT	6-minute walk test
A1AT	alpha-1 antitrypsin deficiency
ABG	arterial blood gas
ABPA	allergic bronchopulmonary aspergillosis
ACE	angiotensin-converting enzyme
ACTH	adrenocorticotropic hormone
ADH	antidiuretic hormone
AFB	acid fast bacilli
AHI	apnoea-hypopnoea index
AIP	acute interstitial pneumonia
ALT	alanine transaminase
ARDS	adult respiratory distress syndrome
ATS	American Thoracic Society
BAL	bronchoalveolar lavage
BCG	Bacille Calmette–Guérin (tuberculosis vaccine)
BCSH	British Committee for Standards in Haematology
BHIVA	British HIV Association
BIPAP	bilevel positive airways pressure
BMI	body mass index
BNP	brain natriuretic peptide
BP	blood pressure
bpm	beats/breaths per minute
BTS	British Thoracic Society
CABG	coronary artery bypass graft
c-ANCA	cytoplasmic antineutrophil cytoplasmic antibody
CAP	community-acquired pneumonia
CF	cystic fibrosis
CFRD	cystic fibrosis-related diabetes
CFT	complement fixation test
CK	creatine kinase
CKD	chronic kidney disease
CMV	Cytomegalovirus
CNS	central nervous system

COP	cryptogenic organizing pneumonia
COPD	chronic obstructive pulmonary disease
CPAP	continuous positive airways pressure
CPX	cardiopulmonary exercise testing
CSF	cerebrospinal fluid
CT	computed tomography (scan)
CTPA	computed tomography pulmonary angiogram
CVID	combined variable immune disorder
CXR	chest X-ray
DAH	diffuse alveolar haemorrhage
DIOS	distal intestinal obstructive syndrome
DIP	desquamative interstitial pneumonia
DM	diabetes mellitus
DOT	directly observed therapy
DPT	diffuse pleural thickening
DVLA	Driver and Vehicle Licensing Agency
DVT	deep vein thrombosis
DEXA	dual-emission X-ray absorptiometry
EBUS	endobronchial ultrasound
EBV	Epstein–Barr virus
ECG	electrocardiogram
ECMO	extracorporeal membrane oxygenation
EPAP	expiratory positive airways pressure
EPTB	extrapulmonary tuberculosis
ERV	expiratory reserve volume
ESC	European Society of Cardiology
ESS	Epworth Sleepiness Score
EUS	endoscopic ultrasound
FBC	full blood count
FEF	forced expiratory flow
FEV_1	forced expiratory volume in 1 second
FNA	fine needle aspiration
FVC	forced vital capacity
GBM	glomerular basement membrane
GBS	Guillian–Barré syndrome
GI	gastrointestinal
GINA	Global Initiative for Asthma
GMC	General Medical Council
GM-CSF	granulocyte-macrophage colony-stimulating factor
GOLD	Global Initiative for Chronic Obstructive Lung Disease

GP	general practitioner
HAART	highly active antiretroviral therapy
Hb	haemoglobin
hCG	human chorionic gonadotropin
HIV	human immunodeficiency virus
HPA	Health Protection Agency
HPS	hepato-pulmonary syndrome
HR	heart rate
HRCT	high-resolution computed tomography
IBD	inflammatory bowel disease
ICU	intensive care unit
Ig	immunoglobulin
IGRA	interferon gamma release assay
ILD	interstitial lung disease
INR	international normalized ratio
IPF	idiopathic pulmonary fibrosis
IPAP	inspiratory positive airways pressure
IRIS	immune reconstitution syndrome
IRV	inspiratory reserve volume
ISWT	incremental shuttle walk test
ITU	intensive therapy unit
IV	intravenous
JRCPTB	Joint Royal Colleges of Physicians Training Board
K^+	potassium
KCO	transfer factor corrected for alveolar volume
LABA	long-acting beta agonist
LAM	lymphangioleiomyomatosis
LAMA	long-acting muscarinic antagonist
LCH	Langerhans cell histiocytosis
LFT	liver function test
LIP	lymphocytic interstitial pneumonia
LN	lymph node
LTB	latent tuberculosis
LTOT	long-term oxygen therapy
LVRS	lung volume reduction surgery
MAC	*Mycobacterium avium* complex
MAI	*Mycobacterium avium-intracellulare*
MC&S	microscopy, culture, and sensitivity
MI	myocardial infarction
MDR	multidrug resistant

MDT	multidisciplinary team
mPAP	mean pulmonary artery pressure
MRI	magnetic resonance imaging (scan)
MTB	Mycobacterium tuberculosis
Na$^+$	sodium
NICE	National Institute of Health and Clinical Excellence
NIV	non-invasive ventilation
NO	nitric oxide
NRT	nicotine replacement therapy
NSAID	non-steroidal anti-inflammatory drug
NSIP	non-specific interstitial pneumonia
NTM	non-tuberculous mycobacterium
NYHA	New York Heart Association
OCP	oral contraceptive pill
OGTT	oral glucose tolerance test
OHS	obesity hypoventilation syndrome
OSA	obstructive sleep apnoea
PA	postero-anterior
p-ANCA	perinuclear antineutrophil cytoplasmic antibody
PAP	pulmonary arterial pressure
PC$_{20}$	provocation concentration
PCD	primary ciliary dyskinesia
PCP	*Pneumocystis* pneumonia
PCR	polymerase chain reaction
PCWP	pulmonary capillary wedge pressure
PE	pulmonary embolism
PEEP	positive end-expiratory pressure
PEFR	peak expiratory flow rate
PET	positive emission tomography
PFT	pulmonary function test
PH	pulmonary hypertension
PLMD	periodic limb movement disorder
PMF	progressive massive fibrosis
ppm	parts per million
prn	as required
PSA	prostate specific antigen
PTB	pulmonary tuberculosis
PTHrP	parathyroid hormone-related protein
QALY	quality-adjusted life year
RA	rheumatoid arthritis

RB	respiratory bronchiolitis
RCOG	Royal College of Obstetricians and Gynaecologists
RCP	Royal College of Physicians
rhDNAse	recombinant human deoxyribonuclease
RLS	restless leg syndrome
RR	respiratory rate
RV	residual volume *or* right ventricle
Sats	oxygen saturations
SBOT	short-burst oxygen therapy
SCE	Specialty Certificate Examination
SIADH	syndrome of inappropriate antidiuretic hormone secretion
SIGN	Scottish Intercollegiate Guidelines Network
SLE	systemic lupus erythematosus
SOB	shortness of breath
TB	tuberculosis
TBLB	transbronchial lung biopsy
TBNA	transbronchial needle aspiration
TLC	total lung capacity
TLCO	total lung carbon monoxide transfer factor
TNF	tumour necrosis factor
TST	tuberculin skin test
TV	tidal volume
U&E	urea and electrolytes
UIP	usual interstitial pneumonia
US	ultrasound
USS	ultrasound scan
VA	alveolar volume
VATS	video-assisted thoracoscopic surgery
VC	vital capacity
V/Q	ventilation/perfusion
WBC	white blood cell
WBP	whole-body plethysmography
WHO	World Health Organization
XDR	extensively drug resistant

1. **A 25 year old man presents to hospital with headache, cough, and chest pain for 4 days. He also describes joint pain and stiffness for 2 days before admission and has noticed a rash over his abdomen and legs. His examination reveals occasional crackles at the right base. His oxygen saturations are 90% on room air. Chest X-ray (CXR) shows bilateral patchy infiltrates. Blood tests are shown in Table 1.1. What is the most likely pathogen?**

Table 1.1 Question 1 - Laboratory results

Test	Result	Normal range
Haemoglobin (Hb)	10.2	11.5–15.0 g/dL
Platelets	110	120–400 × 10^9/L
White blood cell (WBC)	9.2	4–11 × 10^9/L
Sodium (Na^{2+})	130	135–145 mmol/L
Potassium (K^+)	4.6	3.5–5.3 mmol/L
Urea	8	2.5–7.0 mmol/L
Creatinine	92	60–110 mmol/L

A. *Chlamydia psittaci.*
B. *Klebsiella pneumoniae.*
C. *Leigonella pneumophila.*
D. *Mycoplasma pneumoniae.*
E. *Streptococcus pneumoniae.*

2. **A 54 year old man attends your clinic with a 6-month history of dry cough and worsening exertional dyspnoea. He is a smoker with a history of longstanding rheumatoid arthritis (RA), not currently on treatment. Pulmonary function testing demonstrates forced expiratory volume in 1 second (FEV$_1$) 40% predicted, forced vital capacity (FVC) 35% predicted, FEV$_1$:FVC ratio 75%, total lung capacity (TLC) 42% predicted, and transfer factor corrected for alveolar volume (KCO) 15% predicted. Which of the following would be consistent with these findings?**

A. Caplan's syndrome.
B. Pulmonary arterial hypertension.
C. Rheumatoid arthritis-associated interstitial lung disease (RA-ILD).
D. Rheumatoid arthritis-associated pleural effusion.
E. Shrinking lung syndrome.

3. **A 53 year old woman presents with an 8-week history of cough, fever, and sweats. Her blood eosinophil count is 1.0 × 10⁹/L (normal range 0.0–0.4 × 10⁹/L), immunoglobulin E (IgE) is normal. CXR shows bilateral peripheral dense opacification with an inverse pulmonary oedema appearance. Sputum eosinophil count is mildly elevated. What is the most likely diagnosis?**

   A. Acute eosinophilic pneumonia.
   B. Chronic eosinophilic pneumonia.
   C. Churg–Strauss syndrome.
   D. Hypereosinophilic syndrome.
   E. Loeffler's syndrome (simple pulmonary eosinophilia).

4. **A 55 year old woman presents to respiratory clinic with daytime somnolence, impaired concentration, and morning headaches. Her Epworth Sleepiness Score is 12. Full polysomnography demonstrates an apnoea-hypopnoea index of 2 and repetitive limb movements up to 5 seconds in duration, separated by intervals of around 30 seconds. What treatment would you recommend?**

   A. Continuous positive airways pressure (CPAP).
   B. Modafinil.
   C. None.
   D. Paroxetine.
   E. Ropinirole.

5. **A 23 year old man presents with sudden onset shortness of breath and chest pain. He has no significant past medical history. Respiratory rate (RR) is 34/min, saturations 97% breathing room air, and pulse 100 beats per minute (bpm). CXR reveals a 1.8-cm rim of air. What is the most appropriate course of action?**

   A. Admit for high-flow oxygen and repeat CXR in the morning.
   B. Discharge with follow-up CXR in 5 days.
   C. Intercostal drain insertion.
   D. Observe overnight.
   E. Simple aspiration.

6. **A 55 year old man with a body mass index (BMI) of 31 is admitted to hospital. He is known to have chronic obstructive pulmonary disease (COPD) but is normally fully independent. 1 hour after admission, following maximal medical therapy, his blood gas shows pH 7.20, pCO₂ 8.2, pO₂ 8.6 (28% venturi mask), and he is due to be commenced on bilevel positive airways pressure (BIPAP). Which of the following is true regarding the management of this patient?**

   A. He must have a documented resuscitation status in case of BIPAP failure.
   B. He should initially be given a nasal mask in preference to a full face mask.
   C. His pH of 7.20 makes him unsuitable for BIPAP.
   D. Initial BIPAP settings should be inspiratory positive airways pressure (IPAP) 25 and expiratory positive airways pressure (EPAP) 10 cmH₂O.
   E. Oxygen saturations should be maintained at 92–94%.

7. **D-dimer was measured in 200 randomly selected patients with asthma and 200 randomly selected patients with COPD. The data was normally distributed after a logarithmic transformation. Which method of analysis would best identify whether there was a difference between the two groups of patients?**

    A. Chi-square test.
    B. Correlation coefficient.
    C. Logistic regression analysis.
    D. Mann–Whitney U test.
    E. Unpaired T-test.

8. **A 52 year old man presents to the acute assessment unit with a 4-month history of substernal pain and dry cough. His computed tomography (CT) chest is shown in Figure 1.1. What is the likely diagnosis?**

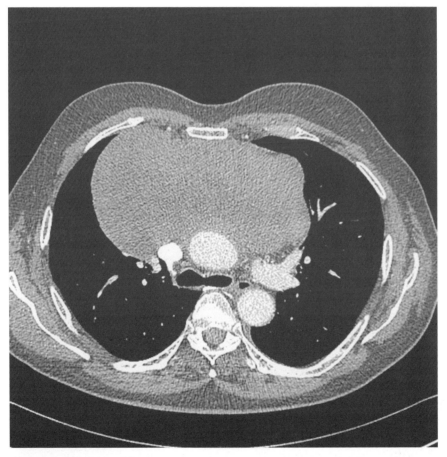

Figure 1.1 Question 8 - CT chest.

A. Aortic aneurysm.
B. Bronchogenic cyst.
C. Retrosternal thyroid goitre.
D. Teratoma.
E. Thymoma.

9. **A 68 year old woman with squamous cell carcinoma of the lung and advanced ischaemic heart disease is reviewed in lung cancer clinic. She is unable to perform strenuous activities, but able to carry out light housework. CT confirms the presence of a tumour of diameter 7 cm, 1.5 cm from the carina, with ipsilateral hilar lymphadenopathy. She has been advised against surgery by her cardiologist. Which of the following treatment modalities is the most appropriate?**

A. Chemotherapy.
B. Lobectomy.
C. Palliative radiotherapy.
D. Radical radiotherapy.
E. Radical radiotherapy plus adjuvant chemotherapy.

10. **You are called to the emergency department to see a 32 year old man admitted with breathlessness and wheeze. He has been treated for acute asthma with steroids and continuous nebulized bronchodilators. His breathing is laboured and he is speaking in short sentences. His RR is 30/min, saturations 94% on 28% oxygen via a venturi mask, pulse 120 bpm, and blood pressure 120/80 mmHg. Arterial blood gas (ABG) demonstrates a metabolic acidosis. Which of the following should you commence now?**

A. High-flow oxygen and close observation.
B. Intravenous (IV) magnesium.
C. IV salbutamol.
D. IV theophylline.
E. Non-invasive ventilation.

11. **A 45 year old man with a 20 pack-year smoking history is referred to clinic with symptoms of worsening exertional dyspnoea. His CT is shown in Figure 1.2. Which of the following diagnoses is most likely?**

A. Asbestosis.
B. Hypersensitivity pneumonitis.
C. Idiopathic pulmonary fibrosis.
D. Sarcoidosis.
E. Non-specific interstitial pneumonia.

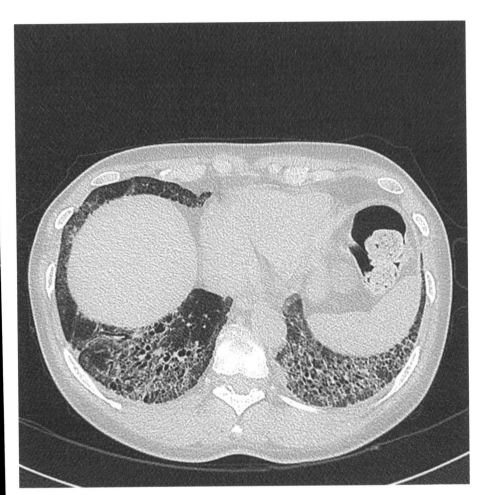

Figure 1.2 Question 11 - CT chest.

12. **You are referred a 30 year old woman who is complaining of shortness of breath. She denies cough or wheeze. She was in a car accident 2 years earlier and was intubated and ventilated on the intensive care unit for 8 weeks. Her flow volume loop and basic spirometry are shown in Figure 1.3 and below. Which is her diagnosis?**

    FVC 4.60 L (100% predicted), FEV$_1$ 2.46 L (67% predicted), FEV$_1$/FVC 53%.

    A. Chest wall deformity.
    B. Post-intubation tracheal stenosis.
    C. Post-ventilation pulmonary fibrosis.
    D. Tracheomalacia.
    E. Vocal cord paralysis.

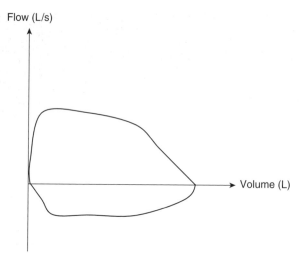

Figure 1.3 Question 12 - Flow volume loop.

13. **You are asked to review a 54 year old woman on the haematology ward. She is 3 weeks post a bone marrow transplant for AML. She has a persistent fever despite broad spectrum antibiotics and a non-productive cough. Her most recent CT scan is shown in Figure 1.4. What is the most likely diagnosis?**

    A. *Aspergillus* infection.
    B. Cavitating bacterial pneumonia.
    C. Cytomegalovirus pneumonia.
    D. *Mycobacterium avium-intracellulare* (MAI).
    E. *Pneumocystis jiroveci* pneumonia (PCP).

14. **A 40 year old female presents to respiratory clinic with symptoms of cough and dyspnoea. She reports a 30 pack-year history of smoking. On auscultation, fine, bibasal end-inspiratory crackles are heard. Pulmonary function tests reveal a mixed obstructive-restrictive pattern with a slightly reduced transfer factor. High-resolution computed tomography (HRCT) demonstrates diffuse ground-glass change and lung biopsy demonstrates pigmented macrophages and mild interstitial inflammatory changes centred around respiratory bronchioles and neighbouring alveoli. How would you manage this patient in the first instance?**

    A. Inhaled steroids.
    B. Oral steroids.
    C. Oral steroids plus azathioprine.
    D. Pulmonary rehabilitation.
    E. Smoking cessation.

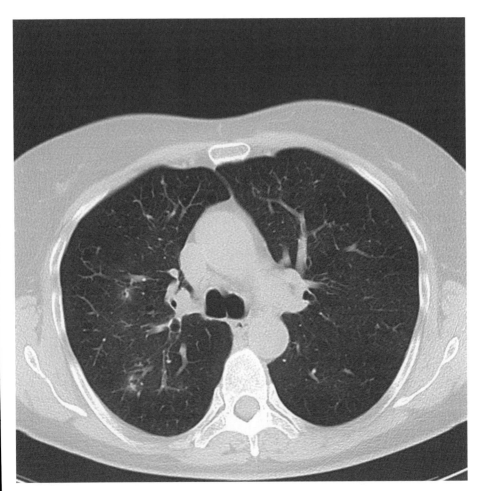

Figure 1.4 Question 13 - CT chest.

15. **A 35 year old woman presents with a 10-day history of cough and fever. She has recently been on holiday to East Africa. On examination she is found to have a temperature of 37.8°C and oxygen saturations of 92% on room air. Blood tests are shown in Table 1.2. Sputum examination reveals eosinophilia and larvae. What is the best treatment?**

    A. Itraconazole.
    B. Mebendazole.
    C. Steroids.
    D. Steroids and itraconazole.
    E. Supportive treatment.

Table 1.2 Question 15 - Laboratory results

Test	Result	Normal range
Hb	13.1	11.5–15.0 g/dL
Platelets	320	120–400 × 10^9/L
WBC	12.0	4–11 × 10^9/L
Neutrophils	8.2	2.0–7.5 × 10^9/L
Eosinophils	1.6	0.0–0.4 × 10^9/L

16. **A 40 year old man attends respiratory clinic with symptoms of snoring, nocturnal choking, daytime somnolence, and impaired sexual function. Polysomnography demonstrates an apnoea-hypopnoea index of 20. He asks you about the implications for his career as a school coach driver. Which of the following is true?**
    A. Falling asleep at the wheel is a criminal offence.
    B. He can drive his car provided he does not feel somnolent.
    C. He will not be able to retain his coach licence and should consider an alternative career.
    D. His general practitioner (GP) can declare him fit to drive his coach once he is established on treatment.
    E. It is the responsibility of the consulting physician to inform the Driver and Vehicle Licensing Agency (DVLA) of his condition.

17. **A 27 year old student, on holiday from New Zealand, presented with a large spontaneous left-sided pneumothorax. It was managed by simple aspiration. Repeat CXR 1 week later shows a very small rim of residual air. He wants to fly home. What should you tell him?**
    A. He can fly immediately.
    B. He can fly 2 weeks after the aspiration.
    C. He can fly 1 week after complete resolution of the pneumothorax.
    D. He needs surgical pleurodesis before flying.
    E. He needs to wait for 6 weeks before flying.

18. **A 66 year old woman is intubated and ventilated for respiratory failure secondary to severe pneumonia. She is heavily sedated. Her ABG after 1 hour of ventilation shows pH 6.9, pCO_2 12, and pO_2 6.2 on 100% oxygen. Her initial ventilator settings are RR 20 breaths per minute (bpm), positive end-expiratory pressure (PEEP) 7.5 cm H_2O, tidal volume (TV) 300 ml. She weights 80 kg. How would you improve her ventilation?**
    A. RR 20, PEEP 10 cm H_2O, TV 600 ml.
    B. RR 30, PEEP 7.5 cm H_2O, TV 300 ml.
    C. RR 25, PEEP 10 cm H_2O, TV 800 ml.
    D. RR 25, PEEP 10 cm H_2O, TV 400 ml.
    E. RR 30, PEEP 5 cm H_2O, TV 400 ml.

19. **A 68 year old man with known COPD attends respiratory clinic with worsening dyspnoea despite maximal medical therapy. Which of the following features would prevent you from offering him lung volume reduction surgery (LVRS)?**

    A. Age >65 years.
    B. FEV_1 30% predicted.
    C. Heterogeneously distributed emphysema.
    D. Pulmonary hypertension.
    E. Total lung carbon monoxide transfer factor (TLCO) >20% predicted.

20. **A 35 year old man presents to clinic with asthma that is poorly controlled on moderate doses of inhaled steroids and recurrent sinusitis. Eosinophilia is demonstrated in peripheral blood and on bronchoalveolar lavage and perinuclear antineutrophil cytoplasmic antibody (p-ANCA) is positive. Surgical lung biopsy confirms a small vessel vasculitis in keeping with Churg–Strauss disease. There is no evidence of extrapulmonary involvement. How should this patient be treated as a first line?**

    A. Methylprednisolone.
    B. Prednisolone.
    C. Steroids plus cyclophosphamide.
    D. Steroids plus azathioprine.
    E. Symptomatically with inhalers.

21. **A patient with breast cancer that is known to have metastasized to the pleura presents with a symptomatic pleural effusion and a complete white-out of her right hemithorax on CXR. She underwent therapeutic aspiration 2 weeks ago with short-lived symptomatic relief. The palliative care team ask you to review her. They estimate she may survive another 3 months. What management would you recommend for her effusion?**

    A. Intercostal drainage.
    B. Intercostal drainage and medical pleurodesis.
    C. No intervention is indicated.
    D. Pleuro-peritoneal shunt.
    E. Repeat therapeutic aspiration.

22. **A 32 year old, non-smoking woman undergoes routine CXR screening for emigration purposes. She has no significant past medical history and is entirely asymptomatic. Her CXR is shown in Figure 1.5. What does the CXR demonstrate?**

    A. Azygous lobe.
    B. Bronchogenic cyst.
    C. Bronchopulmonary sequestration.
    D. Pulmonary agenesis.
    E. Right upper lobe collapse.

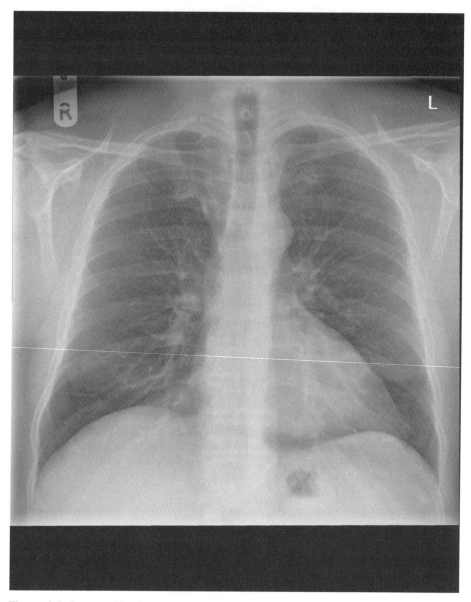

Figure 1.5 Question 22 - Chest radiograph.

23. **A large multicentre randomized controlled trial has been conducted to evaluate the effect of a new lung cancer treatment on 6-month mortality, compared with a placebo. The results are tabulated in Table 1.3. Which statistical method should be used to compare the outcome between the medication and placebo?**

Table 1.3 Question 23 - Study data

	Number alive at 6 months	Number dead at 6 months
New treatment	350	280
Placebo	210	175

A. Chi-square test.
B. Fisher's exact test.
C. Kaplan–Meier analysis.
D. Quality-adjusted life year (QALY) analysis.
E. T-test.

24. **A 54 year old ex-coal miner presents to your clinic with increasing shortness of breath and a non-productive cough. You suspect he has bullous lung disease. Which of the following measurements will help to estimate the volume of bullous disease?**

A. Cardiopulmonary exercise testing.
B. Measurement of lung volumes by helium dilution.
C. Measurement of lung volumes by both helium dilution and whole-body plethysmography.
D. Measurement of lung volumes by whole-body plethysmography.
E. Measurement of TLCO and KCO.

25. **Which of the following statements regarding coal workers' pneumoconiosis is false?**

A. It has no malignant potential.
B. Nodules of Caplan's syndrome are premalignant.
C. Patients with progressive massive fibrosis (PMF) are eligible for compensation.
D. Simple pneumoconiosis does not progress once exposure is removed.
E. The frequency of obstructive disease is increased in coal miners even if they do not smoke.

26. **A 60 year old man with chronic hepatitis and cirrhosis presents with dyspnoea on exertion. Oxygen saturation falls by 7% on sitting up and improves when lying supine. A diagnosis of hepato-pulmonary syndrome (HPS) is suspected. What investigation should be performed to confirm the diagnosis?**

A. Bubble echocardiography using agitated saline.
B. Pulmonary angiography.
C. Pulmonary function testing including transfer factor.
D. Right heart catheterization.
E. Ventilation–perfusion scintigraphy.

27. The relatives of an 80 year old woman with stage IV non-small cell cancer of the lung ask to speak to you on the ward. They inform you that in the event of her further deterioration they wish her to be transferred to the intensive care unit. They pass you a handwritten note, reported to be signed by your patient but not dated or witnessed, which confirms she would also like to be considered for intensive care. What of the following ethical principles are relevant in this case?

    A. Beneficence.
    B. Justice.
    C. Non-maleficence.
    D. Respect for autonomy.
    E. All of the above.

28. A 42 year old male wishes to learn to scuba dive. Which of the following is a contraindication?

    A. Exercise-induced asthma.
    B. Previous treated tuberculosis.
    C. Previous traumatic pneumothorax treated with chest drainage.
    D. Previous spontaneous pneumothorax with bilateral surgical pleurodesis.
    E. Sinusitis.

29. You see a 32 year old woman in clinic who is complaining of worsening shortness of breath on exertion. On examination she is thin with a BMI of 17.5 but with otherwise normal physical examination. She admits to taking fenfluramine in the past. Her pulmonary function tests show: FEV_1 2.0 (125% predicted), FVC 3.0 (79% predicted), FEV_1:FVC 79%, TLCO 52% predicted, KCO 56% predicted, TLC 102% predicted, residual volume (RV) 90% predicted. Which test is most likely to confirm your diagnosis?

    A. Cardiopulmonary exercise testing.
    B. Full blood count.
    C. High-resolution CT scan.
    D. Repeat pulmonary function testing.
    E. Right heart catheterization.

30. A new diagnostic biomarker for pulmonary embolus has been identified. Which of the following parameters measures the proportion of patients with a positive test who have a pulmonary embolism?

    A. Odds ratio.
    B. Positive predictive value.
    C. Relative risk.
    D. Sensitivity.
    E. Specificity.

31. **A 38 year old, non-smoking woman presents to the emergency department with a complete right-sided pneumothorax. She reveals that this is her second pneumothorax and that she previously underwent CT chest, which showed some abnormalities. Her previous CT is available for review (Figure 1.6). Which of the following diagnoses is most likely?**

    A. Alpha-1 antitrypsin deficiency (A1AT) deficiency.
    B. Catamenial pneumothorax.
    C. Langerhans cell histiocytosis (LCH).
    D. Lymphangioleiomyomatosis (LAM).
    E. Pleural bleb rupture.

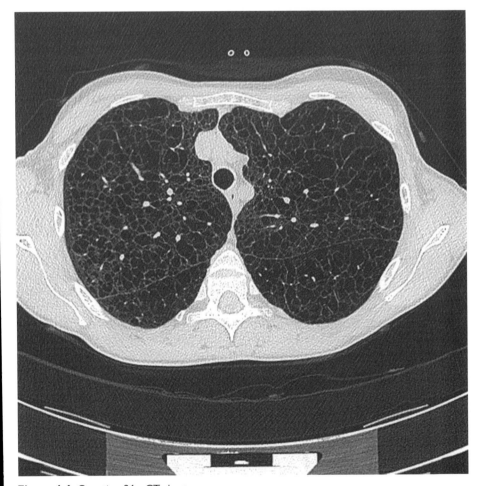

Figure 1.6 Question 31 - CT chest.

32. You see a 43 year old woman in clinic. She was referred by the rheumatologists who are thinking of starting her on anti-tumour necrosis factor (TNF) therapy (infliximab) for her poorly controlled rheumatoid arthritis. She is originally from Southern India but has been in the UK for 14 years. Her CXR shows some small, left apical calcified nodules and apical scarring. She denies any history of tuberculosis (TB) or TB treatment. She is currently on prednisolone 20 mg once daily and has no systemic or respiratory symptoms. What should you do now?

   A. Perform a tuberculin skin test (TST).
   B. Perform an interferon gamma release assay (IGRA).
   C. Repeat the CXR in 3 months.
   D. Start her on treatment for active TB.
   E. Start her on treatment for latent TB.

33. A 47 year old woman complains of mild but worsening shortness of breath, particularly when swimming. She is intermittently breathless at night but this improves with sitting up. Apart from the breathlessness she feels well although her husband reports a slight change in her speech. She has no significant medical history. Her pulmonary function test results demonstrate FEV$_1$ 1.8 L (63% predicted), FVC 2.1 L (61% predicted), FEV$_1$:FVC 86%, RV 1.6 L (115% predicted), TLC 2.49 L (53% predicted), TLCO 89% predicted. Her vital capacity (VC) falls by 22% on lying supine. What is the most likely diagnosis?

   A. Guillain–Barré syndrome.
   B. Hypersensitivity pneumonitis.
   C. Idiopathic pulmonary fibrosis.
   D. Morbid obesity.
   E. Motor neurone disease.

34. A 55 year old man with adenocarcinoma of the lung attends lung cancer clinic to discuss options for surgical resection of the tumour. His CT scan demonstrates a lesion 2 cm in diameter. Positron emission tomography (PET) scanning shows no evidence of suspicious lymphadenopathy or metastatic spread. What adjunctive treatment should you recommend?

   A. None until the surgical outcome has been reviewed.
   B. Preoperative chemotherapy.
   C. Preoperative thoracic radiotherapy.
   D. Postoperative combined chemoradiotherapy.
   E. Prophylactic cranial irradiation.

35. **A 65 year old man with a 40 pack-year history of smoking comes to see you in respiratory clinic with a progressive deterioration in exercise tolerance and exertional wheeze. He tells you he has been diagnosed with asthma. Which of the following makes a diagnosis of chronic asthma more likely than a diagnosis of COPD?**

   A. Airway thickening on CT chest.
   B. Exercise-induced airway hyper-responsiveness.
   C. Increased elastic recoil.
   D. Increased residual volume.
   E. Reduced TLCO.

36. **A 55 year old, morbidly obese woman is diagnosed with severe obstructive sleep apnoea. She describes symptoms of exertional dyspnoea and chest pain. Which of the following would be consistent with a diagnosis of secondary pulmonary hypertension?**

   A. FEV_1:FVC 55% predicted.
   B. Mean pulmonary artery pressure (mPAP) <25 mmHg at rest.
   C. Normal KCO.
   D. Pulmonary capillary wedge pressure (PCWP) >15 mmHg.
   E. Right ventricular dilation and hypokinesis.

37. **A 68 year old man presents with a persistent non-productive cough. He is a retired construction worker with a 30 pack-year smoking history. His CT chest is shown in Figure 1.7. Which of the following diagnoses is the scan most consistent with?**

   A. Bronchogenic malignancy.
   B. Hamartoma.
   C. Metastatic adenocarcinoma.
   D. Pulmonary tuberculosis.
   E. Wegener's granulomatosis.

38. **A 67 year old woman with moderate COPD had a Seldinger chest drain inserted for a large left-sided pneumothorax 3 days ago. She was placed on high-volume, low-pressure wall suction 24 hours ago (−10 cmH$_2$O). She complains of slight discomfort but is otherwise stable. Her CXR today shows resolution of the pneumothorax but the drain continues to swing and bubble. What should you do next?**

   A. Continue with current settings for further 48 hours and review.
   B. Increase the suction pressure to −15 cmH$_2$O.
   C. Refer to thoracic surgeons for consideration of video-assisted thoracoscopic surgery (VATS).
   D. Remove the drain and repeat a CXR.
   E. Replace the Seldinger drain with a large-bore chest tube.

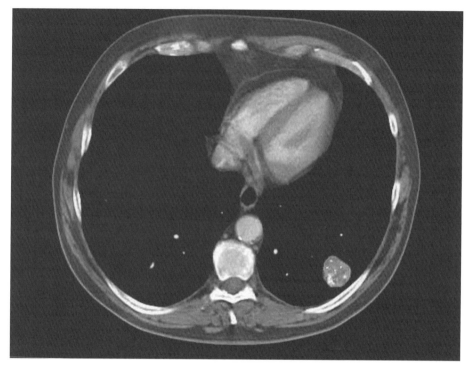

Figure 1.7 Question 37 - CT chest.

39. You see an 18 year old boy with cystic fibrosis in outpatients. He is symptomatically well. His latest sputum culture shows moderate growth of *Pseudomonas aeruginosa*. This is the first time he has grown *Pseudomonas*. Which of the following statements is true?

A. He should attempt *Pseudomonas* eradication with ciprofloxacin and nebulized anti-pseudomonal antibiotics.

B. He should be admitted immediately for 2 weeks of IV anti-pseudomonal antibiotics.

C. He should repeat the sputum culture in 1 month.

D. He should start long-term nebulized anti-pseudomonal antibiotics.

E. No action is needed as he is currently asymptomatic.

40. A young man known to be HIV positive is admitted with pneumonia. His most recent CD4 count is 89. He describes a 3-month history of increasing shortness of breath and cough. He is not sure if he has lost weight. His oxygen saturations drop from 94% to 88% on exertion. CXR is unremarkable. He has been treated with broad-spectrum antibiotics but is not improving. What should you do first?

A. Arrange a bronchoscopy for bronchoalveolar lavage (BAL).

B. Arrange a HRCT chest.

C. Start high-dose antiviral agents.

D. Start treatment for PCP.

E. Start treatment for TB.

41. **A 42 year old businesswoman with a BMI of 35 presents to the acute assessment unit with reduced exercise tolerance. She has a history of atopy and a 25 pack-year smoking history. ABG demonstrates hypoxaemia, hypocapnia, and respiratory alkalosis. Her CXR is shown in Figure 1.8. What is the most likely diagnosis?**
    A. Community-acquired pneumonia.
    B. COPD.
    C. Fat embolism.
    D. Pulmonary hypertension.
    E. Thromboembolism.

42. **A 43 year old man presents to chest clinic with cough, weight loss, and night sweats. The CXR shows apical shadowing on the right. Sputum is smear negative but culture positive for *Mycobacterium tuberculosis*. As part of his screening he had an HIV test that is positive. What should you do?**
    A. Start highly active antiretroviral (HAART) treatment if CD4 <200.
    B. Start HAART now and TB treatment within 2 months.
    C. Start TB treatment and HAART together.
    D. Start TB treatment now and HAART within 2 months.
    E. Treat for TB and start HAART if CD4 < 350.

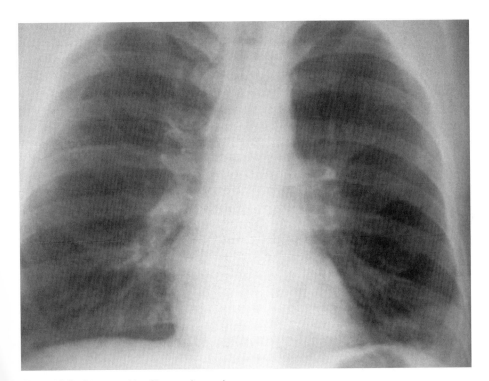

Figure 1.8 Question 41 - Chest radiograph.

43. **A 68 year old woman presents with a 5-day history of low-grade fever, cough, and haemoptysis. Bronchoalveolar lavage results in a haemorrhagic aspirate with haemosiderin-laden macrophages. Her CT chest is shown in Figure 1.9. Which of the following statements is false?**

   A. Diffusing capacity (TLCO) may be increased.
   B. Systemic steroids are the mainstay of treatment.
   C. Repeated haemorrhage may result in irreversible interstitial fibrosis.
   D. The most common histopathological pattern is diffuse alveolar damage.
   E. Pulmonary haemosiderosis is a diagnosis of exclusion.

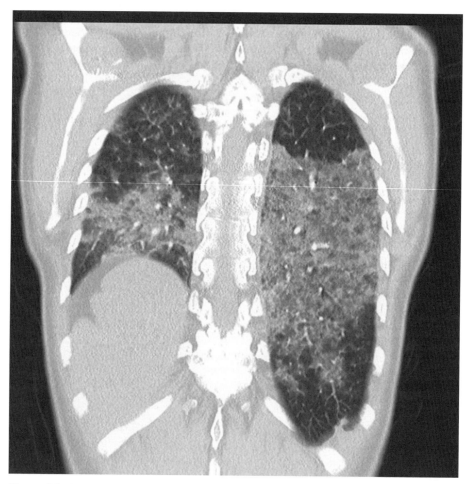

Figure 1.9 Question 43 - CT chest.

44. **A 32 year old woman who is 22 weeks pregnant is travelling to Mexico for a holiday. She is concerned about her risk of contracting swine 'flu. She has heard that pregnant women are especially at risk. What should you advise her?**

    A. Immunization is associated with teratogenicity in the second trimester.
    B. She should be immunized against swine 'flu.
    C. She should not travel to Mexico.
    D. She should take oseltamivir (Tamiflu) with her in case she develops symptoms.
    E. The pandemic is over so there is no need to be concerned.

45. **A randomized controlled trial has been established to compare the efficacy of a new inhaled medication against placebo in the treatment of asthma. The results suggest there is no statistical difference in efficacy between the medication and placebo. A statistician suggests the results may represent a type II error. What is the implication of this?**

    A. Inappropriate statistical tests were used.
    B. The p value was miscalculated.
    C. The results were affected by observer bias.
    D. The results were affected by interpretation bias.
    E. The study was too small to detect a statistical difference between treatments.

46. **A 65 year old former shipbuilder with known ankylosing spondylitis and a 50 pack-year smoking history presents with shortness of breath on exertion. Pulmonary function tests demonstrate a restrictive defect. His CT chest is shown in Figure 1.10. What is the most likely diagnosis?**

    A. Diffuse pleural thickening.
    B. Mesothelioma.
    C. Metastatic adenocarcinoma.
    D. Pleural plaque disease.
    E. Shrinking pleuritis.

47. **A 29 year old woman attends cystic fibrosis clinic with an increasing frequency of exacerbations, one of which required recent admission to intensive care. She reports deterioration in exercise tolerance and pulmonary function tests demonstrate a rapid decline in FEV$_1$ to 25% predicted. Which of the following is an absolute contraindication to lung transplantation?**

    A. BMI <15 kg/m^2.
    B. Colonization with mucoid *Pseudomonas aeruginosa* and *Burkholderia cepacia*.
    C. Poor compliance with prescribed medication.
    D. Previous pleurectomy.
    E. Recent mechanical ventilation.

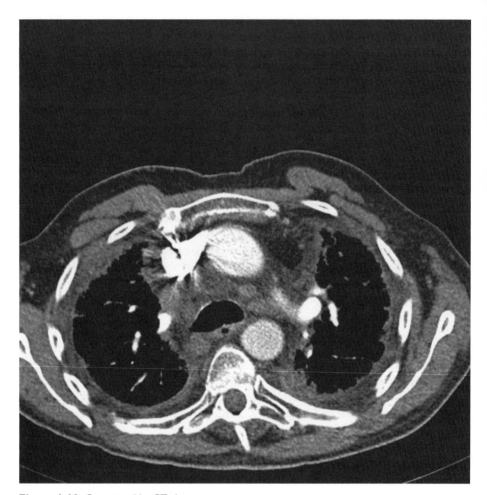

Figure 1.10 Question 46 - CT chest.

48. **You see a 55 year old woman in the chest clinic. She complains of several months of weight loss, productive cough, progressive lethargy and shortness of breath. She has had a CXR which shows right middle lobe patchy consolidation and some bronchiectasis in the right upper lobe and lingula. She has already submitted a sputum sample and *Mycobacterium avium-intracellulare* has been cultured. What is the next step in her management?**

   A. A further positive sputum culture before treatment.

   B. Bronchoscopy for biopsy samples before treatment.

   C. 2HRZE 4HR.

   D. 12HE.

   E. 24HE.

49. A 70 year old woman presents to clinic with a 1-month history of unexplained weight loss, worsening shortness of breath, and dry cough with intermittent small volume haemoptysis. A CXR taken by her GP 3 weeks ago was unremarkable. Her current CXR is shown in Figure 1.11. Which of the following diagnoses is the CXR most consistent with?

    A. Bronchoalveolar cell carcinoma.

    B. Congestive cardiac failure.

    C. Lymphangitis carcinomatosis.

    D. Lymphoma.

    E. Sarcoidosis.

50. A 32 year old male complains of recurrent cough and sputum production. He reports multiple lower respiratory tract infections and he remembers being treated for recurrent ear infections as a child. On examination he is thin and clubbed and has occasional crackles in the middle zones bilaterally. His oxygen saturations are 94% on room air. On further questioning he admits he and his wife have been trying for a baby for some time without success. What is the most likely diagnosis?

    A. A1AT deficiency.

    B. Combined variable immune disorder (CVID).

    C. Cystic fibrosis.

    D. Primary ciliary dyskinesia.

    E. Post-pertussis bronchiectasis.

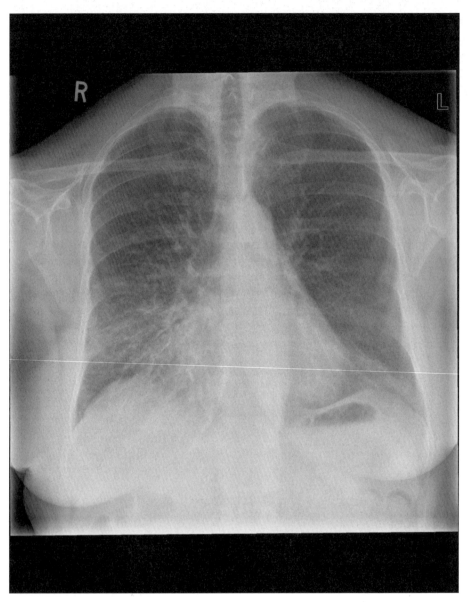

Figure 1.11 Question 49 - Chest radiograph.

OBSTRUCTIVE LUNG DISEASE

Asthma

Diagnosis

- Features: wheeze, breathlessness, chest tightness and cough, typically worse at night, exacerbated by allergen exposure, extremes of temperature and exercise.
  - If history and examination suggest either a high probability of asthma or an intermediate probability of asthma with $FEV_1:FVC <0.7$, commence treatment.
  - If the diagnosis is uncertain and $FEV_1:FVC >0.7$, arrange investigation.
- Investigation:
  - Peak expiratory flow rate (PEFR): diurnal variation >20%; improvement post bronchodilator $\geq 20\%$ or >60 L/min.
  - Spirometry: 400 ml increase in FEV_1 post bronchodilator or after steroid trial (prednisolone 30 mg daily for 14 days).
  - Bronchial stimulation (methacholine/histamine): $PC_{20} <8$ mg/ml, where PC_{20} is the provocative concentration that results in a 20% fall in FEV_1.
  - Other: sputum eosinophilia >2% and exhaled nitric oxide (NO) >50 ppb suggest eosinophilic airway inflammation and potential steroid responsiveness.

Differential diagnoses

- Hyperventilation, vocal cord dysfunction, laryngeal disease, foreign body, malignancy, COPD, obliterative bronchiolitis.

Symptom control

- Asthma is well controlled if there are no daytime symptoms, no night-time awakening due to asthma, no need for rescue medication, no exacerbations, no limitations on activity including exercise, and FEV_1 and/or PEFR exceeds 80% predicted/best.
- Control may deteriorate as a result of smoking, environmental factors, psychosocial factors, poor inhaler technique, poor compliance with medication, chronic rhinosinusitis, allergic bronchopulmonary aspergillosis (ABPA), bronchiectasis, or gastro-oesophageal reflux.

Management of stable asthma

- General measures: weight reduction if obese, smoking cessation, Buteyko breathing technique (control of hyperventilation).
- Step 1: inhaled short-acting β2 agonist as required (prn).
- Step 2: add inhaled steroid 200–800 mcg/day.
- Step 3: add inhaled long-acting β agonist (LABA). If control remains inadequate, increase inhaled steroid to 800 mcg/day and consider trial of leukotriene antagonist or slow-release theophylline *or* consider budesonide/formoterol combination inhaler for regular and rescue use.

- Step 4: increase inhaled steroid to 2000 mcg/day and add fourth agent, e.g. leukotriene antagonist, slow-release theophylline, or oral β2 agonist.
- Step 5: maintain high-dose inhaled steroid and add daily prednisolone at lowest dose for control.
- Step down: Review every 3 months and aim to reduce steroid dose by 25–50%.

Reference: British Thoracic Society/ Scottish Intercollegiate Guidelines Network 2011.

Immunotherapy

- May be considered if a clinically significant allergen cannot be avoided.
- Risk of severe allergic reaction to therapy.

Anti-IgE therapy (Omalizumab)

- Indications:
  - Severe, persistent, allergic asthma.
  - Confirmed IgE-mediated allergy to perennial allergen; IgE level 30–700 IU/mL.
  - Symptoms despite compliance with maximal inhaled therapy and oral steroids.
  - ≥2 exacerbations requiring hospital admission in the preceding year or ≥3 severe exacerbations requiring monitoring in an emergency department with at least 1 admission to hospital.
- Should be supervised by a physician experienced in both allergy and respiratory medicine in a specialist centre.
- Discontinue at 16 weeks if there is no adequate response to therapy.

Reference: National Institute of Health and Clinical Excellence Guidelines 2007.

Acute asthma

- Moderate: PEFR 50–75% predicted/best.
- Acute severe: PEFR 33–50% predicted/best, HR ≥110/min, RR ≥25/min, inability to complete a sentence in a single breath.
- Life threatening: PEFR <33% predicted/best; SpO_2 <92%, PaO_2 <8 kPa; normal $PaCO_2$ (4.6–6.0 kPa); silent chest; cyanosis; poor respiratory effort; arrhythmia; altered conscious state.
- Near fatal: raised $PaCO_2$; requirement for mechanical ventilation with raised inflation pressures.

Management of acute asthma

- Admit any patient with features of an acute severe attack persisting after treatment, or any features of a life-threatening or near fatal attack. Discharge patients whose PEFR is >75% predicted/best 1 hr after initial treatment.
- Give supplementary oxygen to maintain SpO_2 94–98%.
- β2 agonists: high-dose inhaled β2 agonists recommended as a first line; use oxygen-driven nebulizers if there are features of life-threatening asthma or a poor response to inhaled therapy.
- Ipratropium bromide: recommended for patients with a poor response to β2 agonists or features of severe/life-threatening asthma.
- Steroids: recommended for all patients—prednisolone 40–50 mg daily for ≥5 days.
- Magnesium sulphate: give a single IV dose in patients with a poor response to bronchodilators or features of severe/life-threatening asthma.
- Other: aminophylline should not be used in addition to high-dose β2 agonists, but may be useful if there are no β2 agonists available. Antibiotics and adrenaline should not be used routinely.

Intensive care in acute asthma

- Refer any patient with features of: PEFR deteriorating despite therapy, persisting or worsening hypoxia, hypercapnia, acidosis on ABG analysis, exhaustion/poor respiratory effort, altered conscious level, respiratory arrest.

Exercise-induced asthma

- An expression of poorly controlled asthma.
- In addition to regular steroid inhalers consider a leukotriene antagonist, LABA, oral β2 agonist, chromones or slow-release theophylline.
- Advise short-acting β2 agonists immediately prior to exercise.

Asthma in pregnancy

- Most asthma medications are safe during pregnancy.
- Leukotriene antagonists may be continued in women in whom they have proven benefit but are not routinely started during pregnancy.
- Acute severe asthma in pregnancy is an emergency and should be managed the same as in the non-pregnant patient, with continuous fetal monitoring.
- Acute asthma during labour is rare and normal vaginal delivery should be attempted.
- Regular medication should be continued. Women receiving prednisolone at a dose ≥7.5 mg per day for ≥2 weeks prior to delivery should be given hydrocortisone at a dose of 100 mg 6–8-hrly.

Occupational asthma

- See Chapter 12: Occupational and environmental lung diseases.

Alpha-1 antitrypsin deficiency (A1AT)

- Affects 1:3000 in the UK and accounts for 1–3% of newly diagnosed COPD.
- Failure to inhibit the action of the protease neutrophil elastase:
  - Early onset emphysema (lower lobe), bronchiectasis.
  - Chronic hepatitis ± cirrhosis, increased risk of hepatocellular carcinoma.
- An autosomal co-dominant disorder of the *SERPINA1* (Pi) gene; chromosome 14:
  - Multiple genotypes: PiMM (normal), MZ, MS, SS, SZ, ZZ.
  - PiMZ, PiMS, PiSS: 60–80% of normal serum level; not always pathological.
  - PiSZ: 40% of normal serum level; emphysema common.
  - PiZZ: 10% of normal serum level; severe variant with lung and liver disease.
- Normal serum level of A1AT is 20–53 μmol/L; levels above 11 μmol/L are protective.
- Investigation: plasma electrophoresis, A1AT levels, genotypic studies.
- Management: smoking cessation, alcohol restriction (limited evidence), supportive treatment, recombinant A1AT (not recommended by NICE), genetic counselling.

Chronic obstructive pulmonary disease (COPD)

Diagnosis

- Clinical: exertional dyspnoea, chronic cough, regular sputum production, wheeze.

- Investigation:
  - Spirometry: FEV_1:FVC ratio <0.7, obstruction not fully reversible.
  - ± serial pulmonary function tests including TLCO, CT thorax, electrocardiogram (ECG)/ echocardiography (ECHO) for cor pulmonale, ABG for long-term oxygen therapy assessment, sputum culture.

Classification of COPD (with FEV_1:FVC <70)

- Stage 1: mild—FEV_1 ≥80% predicted.
- Stage 2: moderate—FEV_1 50–79% predicted.
- Stage 3: severe—FEV_1 30–49% predicted.
- Stage 4: very severe—FEV_1 <30% predicted.

Reference: National Institute of Health and Clinical Excellence Guidelines 2010.

Exacerbation of COPD

- Defined as a sustained worsening of symptoms which is acute in onset.
- Routine investigations must include CXR, ABG, ECG, full blood count (FBC), urea and electrolytes (U&Es), theophylline level if taking methylxanthines, sputum culture if purulent, blood culture if pyrexial.
- If inhaled bronchodilators are ineffective, use air-driven nebulizers.
- IV theophylline should only be used if there is an inadequate response to nebulizers.
- Commence prednisolone 30 mg daily for 7–14 days.
- Non-invasive ventilation recommended for persistent hypercapnic respiratory failure.

Management of stable COPD

- First-line therapy is empirical short-acting β2 agonists:
  - If FEV_1 ≥ 50% predicted: add LABA or long-acting muscarinic antagonist (LAMA).
  - If FEV_1 < 50% predicted: add LABA plus inhaled steroid (via combination inhaler) or LAMA.
  - If control remains poor, offer LAMA in addition to LABA and inhaled steroid, irrespective of FEV_1.
- Theophylline should only be used after a trial of short- and long-acting bronchodilators in patients unable to use inhaled therapy. Reduce dose if concurrent macrolides/fluoroquinolones are prescribed.
- Consider nebulized therapy in patients with persistent symptoms despite maximal inhaled therapy.
- Oral steroids should not be prescribed for routine maintenance. Patients on long-term steroids aged >65 years should receive osteoporosis prophylaxis.
- Pneumococcal vaccination and an annual influenza vaccination should be offered.
- Antioxidant therapy, antitussives, and prophylactic antibiotics are not recommended.

Reference: National Institute of Health and Clinical Excellence Guidelines 2010.

Surgical intervention

- Bullectomy: if symptomatic, single large bulla on CT and FEV_1 <50% predicted.
- Lung volume reduction surgery (LVRS): if FEV_1 20–45% predicted, $PaCO_2$ <7.3 kPa, heterogenous emphysema and TLCO >20% predicted.
- Transplant: for very severe/progressive disease.

Smoking cessation

- Interventional elements: opportunistic advice, individual and group behaviour therapy, self-help materials, and support services.
- Pharmacotherapy:
  - Nicotine replacement therapy (NRT), bupropion (a noradrenaline-dopamine reuptake inhibitor), and varenicline (a partial agonist of the $\alpha4\beta2$ nicotinic acetylcholine receptor) have proven beneficial effects.
  - Do not use NRT, bupropion, or varenicline in any combination.
  - NRT, bupropion, and varenicline may be used with caution in patients with unstable cardiovascular disease.
  - Bupropion and varenicline should not be offered to patients aged <18 years, pregnant or breastfeeding.
  - Bupropion lowers seizure threshold and is contraindicated in epileptics.
- Success is validated by a CO monitor reading <10 ppm at 4 weeks.

Pulmonary rehabilitation

- An individualized programme of exercise training, education, behavioural therapy, and outcome assessment. Ideally ≥2 supervised sessions per week for ≥6 weeks.
- Contraindications: patients unable to walk, with unstable angina or recent myocardial infarction (MI).
- Benefits: reduced re-admission rates in COPD, improved exercise tolerance (measured by 6-minute walk (6MWT)/shuttle walk test), reduced sensation of dyspnoea, and improved health-related quality of life. There are no proven benefits on lung function or mortality.
- Benefits are partially maintained for around 1 year then diminish.

Home oxygen

- Short-burst oxygen therapy (SBOT):
  - For symptomatic relief of dyspnoea if all other methods fail.
  - Apparent benefits may be due to cooling effect of oxygen on the face; similar effect with fan therapy.
- Long-term oxygen therapy (LTOT):
  - Assessment: ABG on 2 occasions ≥3 weeks apart. Patient must be clinically stable and on optimum medical management.
  - Indications:
    - PaO_2 < 7.3kPa.
    - PaO_2 7.3–8.0kPa with any of:
      - secondary polycythaemia: haematocrit > 55%
      - nocturnal hypoxaemia: SaO_2 <90% for >30% of the time
      - peripheral oedema
      - pulmonary hypertension.
    - Terminally ill patients who require palliation.
  - Oxygen should be used for ≥15 hrs and ideally >20 hrs per day for mortality benefit in COPD.
  - Smoking is not an absolute contraindication but patients should be warned about the risk of fire/explosion.

Ambulatory oxygen

- For patients on LTOT who wish to continue oxygen therapy outside the home.
- For patients with exercise desaturation with demonstrated improvement in exercise capacity or relief of dyspnoea symptoms with oxygen.

THORACIC ONCOLOGY AND PALLIATIVE CARE

Thoracic oncology

Types of lung cancer

- Small cell (15%).
- Non-small cell (85%):
  - ◆ Adenocarcinoma (35–40% of total).
  - ◆ Squamous cell (25–30%).
  - ◆ Large cell (10–15%).
  - ◆ Bronchoalveolar cell carcinoma (2–3%).
  - ◆ Carcinoid (1%).

Paraneoplastic syndromes

- Small cell:
  - ◆ Syndrome of inappropriate antidiuretic hormone secretion (SIADH), ectopic adrenocortico-tropic hormone (ACTH) (Cushing's syndrome), Eaton–Lambert myasthenic syndrome, cerebellar syndrome, limbic encephalitis.
- Non-small cell:
  - ◆ Adenocarcinoma: clubbing, hypertrophic pulmonary osteoarthropathy, Trousseau's syndrome of hypercoagulability.
  - ◆ Squamous cell: hypercalcaemia (parathyroid hormone-related protein (PTHRP) production).

Superior vena cava obstruction

- Most commonly due to lung cancer, especially small cell, and lymphoma.
- Investigation:
  - ◆ CXR/contrast-enhanced CT.
  - ◆ Obtain tissue diagnosis prior to treatment unless there is laryngeal oedema/stridor.
- Management:
  - ◆ Immediate: oxygen, sit up, analgesia ± steroids.
  - ◆ Subsequent:
    - ▪ Small cell and lymphoma: chemotherapy ± intraluminal stent.
    - ▪ Non-small cell: radiotherapy ± intraluminal stent.

Investigation of suspected lung cancer

- Indications for urgent CXR:
  - ◆ Haemoptysis.
  - ◆ If unexplained or lasting >3 weeks:
    - ▪ Symptoms: hoarseness, cough, thoracic pain, dyspnoea, weight loss.
    - ▪ Signs: chest signs, finger clubbing, lymphadenopathy, metastases.

- If malignancy suspected, perform contrast-enhanced CT chest/liver/adrenals.
- Peripheral/central lesion:
  - Low probability of mediastinal malignancy—peripheral lesion, nodes <10 mm:
    - Curative intent: PET-CT.
    - Non-curative intent: transthoracic needle biopsy.
  - Intermediate probability of mediastinal malignancy—nodes 10–20 mm.
    - Any of PET-CT, endobronchial ultrasound transbronchial needle aspiration (EBUS TBNA), endoscopic ultrasound fine needle aspiration (EUS FNA), non-US TBNA.
    - ± Surgical staging.
    - Evaluate PET positive nodes by mediastinal sampling.
  - High probability of mediastinal malignancy—nodes >20 mm:
    - US-guided neck node biopsy or non-US TBNA.
    - If negative, follow with EBUS TBNA, EUS FNA, non-US TBNA.
    - ± Surgical staging.
- Central lesion where staging does not affect treatment:
  - Bronchoscopy plus non-US TBNA.
  - If negative, follow with EBUS TBNA, EUS FNA.
  - ± Surgical staging.
- Neck nodes:
  - US-guided neck node biopsy.
  - If negative, follow with EBUS TBNA, EUS FNA, non-US TBNA.
  - ± Surgical staging.
- Metastatic disease:
  - PET-CT/magnetic resonance imaging (MRI) plus biopsy of most accessible site.

Reference: National Institute of Health and Clinical Excellence Guidelines 2011.

Lung cancer staging

Non-small cell

- TNM staging
  - Tumour:
    - T0: no evidence of primary tumour.
    - T1:
      - T1a: tumour diameter <2 cm.
      - T1b: tumour diameter 2–3 cm.
    - T2:
      - T2a: tumour diameter 3–5 cm.
      - T2b: tumour diameter 5–7 cm.
      - Or: tumour in the main bronchus >2 cm from the carina, invasion of the visceral pleura or localized atelectasis/pneumonitis.
    - T3:
      - Tumour diameter >7 cm.
      - Or: tumour invading any of the chest wall, diaphragm, mediastinal pleura, parietal pericardium, tumour in the main bronchus within 2 cm but not involving the carina, tumour associated with atelectasis/pneumonitis of the entire lung.
      - Or: more than one tumour nodule in the same lobe of the lung.

- T4:
  - Tumour of any size.
  - Tumour invading the mediastinum, heart, great vessels, oesophagus, trachea, carina, vertebral body.
  - *Or:* tumour nodules in more than one lobe of the same lung.
- Regional lymph nodes:
  - N0: no evidence of regional lymph node metastases.
  - N1: Metastases to ipsilateral peribronchial/perihilar lymph nodes; intrapulmonary nodes related to direct tumour extension.
  - N2: Metastases to ipsilateral mediastinal/subcarinal lymph nodes.
  - N3: Contralateral or supraclavicular lymph nodes.
- Distant metastases:
  - M0: no distant metastases.
  - M1:
    - M1a: malignant pleural or pericardial effusion.
    - M1b: distant metastases present.

Reference: Union for International Cancer Control Guidelines 2009.

- Stage grouping by TNM subsets

Table 3.1 Stage grouping by TNM subsets

Stage	Tumour	Lymph nodes	Metastases	5-year survival
IA	T1a or T1b	N0	M0	61%
IB	T2a	N0	M0	38%
IIA	T1a or T1b or T2a	N1	M0	34%
	T2b	N0	M0	
IIB	T2b	N1	M0	24%
	T3	N0	M0	
IIIA	T1a–T3	N2	M0	13%
	T3	N1	M0	
	T4	N0 or N1	M0	
IIIB	T4	N2	M0	5%
	T1a–T4	N3	M0	
IV	Any T	Any N	M1a or M1b	1%

Reference: Union for International Cancer Control Guidelines 2009.

Small cell

- TNM system rarely used.
- Disease classified as limited or extensive:
  - Limited: confined to the ipsilateral thorax and contralateral mediastinal/supraclavicular nodes.
  - Extensive: metastases in the contralateral lung or distant metastases.

Management

Non-small cell

- Offer radical treatment to patients with T1a–3 N0–1 M0 disease:
  - Radical surgery is first-line option.
  - Radical radiotherapy indicated for:
    - patients with early stage lung cancer and high surgical risk
    - patients who choose not to have surgery.
- Radical surgery:
  - Open or thoracoscopic lobectomy is preferred.
  - Limited resection:
    - Indicated in small tumours (T1a–b N0 M0) and borderline fitness.
    - Segmentectomy, wedge resection.
  - Extensive resection:
    - Indicated only to obtain clear margins.
    - Bi-lobectomy, pneumonectomy, bronchoangioplastic surgery.
  - Perform lymph node sampling or en bloc resection in all patients.
  - Contraindications:
    - Absolute: MI within 30 days.
    - Relative: ≥3 cardiac risk factors, active cardiac condition, angina requiring revascularization, poor cardiac function, FEV1 or TLCO <30% predicted, VO2max <15 ml/kg/min, shuttle walk <400 m.
  - Preoperative chemotherapy or radiotherapy not recommended.
  - Postoperative chemotherapy may be offered as adjuvant therapy:
    - Performance status WHO 0–1.
    - Plus T1–3 N1–2 M0 or T2–3 N0 M0 with tumour >4 cm diameter.
  - Consider postoperative radiotherapy only if resection margins are not clear.
- Radical radiotherapy:
  - Performance status WHO 0–1.
  - Disease limited to a radiotherapy treatment volume which will not result in unacceptable damage to healthy tissue.
  - Radiotherapy options:
    - Continuous hyperfractionated accelerated radiotherapy (CHART).
    - Conventional fractionated radiotherapy: 64–66 Gy in 32–33 fractions over 6.5 weeks or 55 Gy in 20 fractions over 4 weeks.
  - Offer concurrent or sequential chemoradiotherapy for locally advanced (stage II/III) disease.
- Chemotherapy alone:
  - Stage III or IV disease; performance status WHO 0–1 or Karnofsky 80–100.
  - No curative effect.
  - Chemotherapy options:
    - Combination of a 3rd-generation agent (docetaxel, gemcitabine, paclitaxel) plus a platinum drug (carboplatin, cisplatin).
    - Single agent docetaxel as second-line therapy.
- Symptomatic treatment:
  - Endobronchial obstruction: radiotherapy, debulking surgery, stenting.
  - Brain metastases: whole brain radiotherapy if symptomatic metastases and WHO 0–1, dexamethasone titrated to symptoms.
  - Bone metastases: standard analgesia, single fraction radiotherapy.
  - Malignant effusion: aspiration or drainage, pleurodesis.

Reference: National Institute of Health and Clinical Excellence, 2011/ British Thoracic Society Guidelines 2010.

Small cell

- Surgery:
  - ◆ Limited disease with no nodal involvement or metastases may be amenable to surgical resection as part of multimodality management.
- Combined chemoradiotherapy:
  - ◆ Limited disease:
    - Multidrug, cisplatin based (carboplatin if renal impairment, WHO ≥2 or significant comorbidity); 4–6 cycles if responsive.
    - WHO 0–1: concurrent radical radiotherapy; start during 1st/2nd chemotherapy cycle.
    - WHO >1: radical radiotherapy within 6 weeks of completion of chemotherapy.
  - ◆ Extensive disease:
    - Platinum-based combination chemotherapy.
    - Thoracic radiotherapy after chemotherapy in patients with complete response to chemotherapy at distal sites and partial chest response.
- Prophylactic cranial irradiation recommended in patients with WHO 0–2 who respond to first-line treatment.
- Second-line chemotherapy only if disease responded to first line.

Reference: National Institute of Health and Clinical Excellence, 2011/ British Thoracic Society Guidelines 2010.

Nodules detected during non-screening CT chest

(Considering smokers as high risk)
- ◆ ≤4 mm (<1% malignant):
  - Low risk: discharge.
  - High risk: CT at 12 months, discharge if unchanged.
- ◆ 4–6 mm:
  - Low risk: CT at 12 months, discharge if unchanged.
  - High risk: CT at 6–12 months and 18–24 months if unchanged.
- ◆ 6–8 mm:
  - Low risk: CT at 6–12 months and 18–24 months if unchanged.
  - High risk: CT at 3–6 months, 9–12 months, and 24 months if unchanged.
- ◆ 8 mm:
  - Low and high risk: CT at 3 months, 9 months and 24 months; consider PET/biopsy/ excision.

Reference: Fleischner Society Guidelines 2005.

Palliative care

- The active total care of patients whose disease is not responsive to curative treatment.

Liverpool Care Pathway

- Recommended by the Department of Health as the best practice model for care of the dying.

- Indications:
  - Multidisciplinary team (MDT) agree patient is dying.
  - Plus 2 or more of bed-bound, semi-comatose, only able to take sips of fluid, no longer able to take tablets.
- Staff are pre-authorized to give interventions/medication to address:
  - Pain: morphine/diamorphine.
  - Agitation: midazolam.
  - Respiratory tract secretions: hyoscine hydrobromide/glycopyrronium.
  - Nausea and vomiting: cyclizine/haloperidol/levomepromazine.
  - Shortness of breath: midazolam/diamorphine.

Advance directives

- Individuals have the right to refuse treatment but not to demand treatment deemed inappropriate or illegal (e.g. assisted suicide).
- Conditions for validity of advance directives:
  - Completed voluntarily whilst the patient has capacity.
  - The patient is >18 years old.
  - The patient has a full understanding of the medical implications if the directive is respected.
  - In writing, signed, dated, and witnessed.
  - Applicable to the patient's present circumstances.
- Legal status:
  - Valid and applicable advance directives are legally binding in England and Wales but have yet to be tested in the courts in Scotland and Northern Ireland.
  - Advance directives are legitimized in the Mental Capacity Act (2005).
- Lasting power of attorney (LPA):
  - Advance directives cannot be used to entrust treatment decisions to another individual.
  - LPA is a legal document appointing an individual responsible for decision-making when the subject lacks the mental capacity to do so themselves.

PULMONARY INFECTION

Pneumonia

Definitions

- Community-acquired pneumonia (CAP): occurs within 48 hrs of admission.
- Hospital-acquired pneumonia: occurs ≥48 hrs after admission.
- Ventilator-acquired pneumonia: occurs ≥48 hrs after intubation.

Severity assessment

CURB-65 score

- Each risk factor scores 1 point: confusion of new onset (AMT ≤8), urea ≥7 mmol/L, respiratory rate ≥30 breaths per minute, blood pressure <90 mmHg systolic or <60 mmHg diastolic, age ≥65 years.
- Mortality increases with CURB-65 score:
    - 0–1: <3%.
    - 2: 9%.
    - 3–5: 15–40%.
- Interpretation:
    - 0–1: Low severity - treat as an outpatient.
    - 2: Moderate severity - close observation ± short hospital admission.
    - 3–5: High severity - requires hospital admission ± high dependency care.

Microbiology: commonly diagnosed pathogens

- Community-acquired pneumonia:
    - Most commonly: *Streptococcus pneumoniae*, *Mycoplasma pneumoniae*, *Chlamydia pneumoniae*, and respiratory viruses.
    - Less commonly: *Legionella pneumoniae*, *Haemophilus influenza*.
- Hospital-acquired pneumonia:
    - MRSA, MSSA, Gram-negative bacteria (*Pseudomonas*, *Klebsiella*, *Enterobacter*, *Escherichia coli*, *Acinetobacter*, *Proteus*).
- Ventilator-associated pneumonia:
    - MRSA, MSSA, Gram-negative bacteria (*Pseudomonas*, *Acinetobacter*, *Stenotrophomonas maltophilia*).
- Aspiration pneumonia:
    - 40% of healthy individuals have nocturnal microaspiration.
    - Chemical pneumonitis, bacterial infection, or both.
    - Gram-negative anaerobes (*Peptostreptococcus*, *Prevotella*, *Bacteroides*, *Fusobacterium*) and mixed infection common.

- Cavitating pneumonia/abscess formation:
  - *Streptococcus milleri*, *Staphylococcus aureus*, *Klebsiella*, *Streptococcus pyogenes*, *H. influenzae*, *Legionella*, *Nocardia*, *Actinomyces*, *Mycobacterium tuberculosis* (thick walled).
  - Multiple abscesses: *S. aureus*, septic emboli.
  - Immunocompromised: *Pseudomonas*, *Nocardia*, PCP, fungi (*Aspergillus/Cryptococcus/Histoplasma*).
- Atypical pathogens:
  - *Mycoplasma*, *Chlamydia pneumonia/psittaci*, *Coxiella burnetii* (*not Legionella* as per BTS).

Special patient groups

- Alcoholic patients:
  - Increased risk of aspiration and cavity formation.
  - *S. pneumoniae* (often with bacteraemia), Gram-negative bacteria (especially *Klebsiella*), *Legionella* and atypical infections more common.
- COPD patients:
  - *H. influenzae* and *M. catarrhalis* more common.
- Diabetic patients:
  - *S. pneumoniae* with bacteraemia more common
- Elderly patients:
  - *S. pneumoniae* more common; *Mycoplasma* and *Legionella* less common

Antibiotic management

- Always check local antibiotic guidelines.
- Empirical therapy:
  - Low severity:
    - Oral antibiotics: amoxicillin or doxycycline if penicillin intolerant.
  - Moderate severity:
    - Oral antibiotics if possible.
    - Amoxicillin plus macrolide (clarithromycin).
    - If penicillin intolerant: doxycycline, moxifloxacin, levofloxacin.
    - IV antibiotics if oral not tolerated: amoxicillin or benzylpenicillin plus clarithromycin.
    - IV and penicillin intolerant: levofloxacin monotherapy or cephalosporin plus macrolide.
  - High severity:
    - Rapid administration of IV antibiotics.
    - Augmentin plus macrolide or cephalosporin plus macrolides.
- Antibiotic duration:
  - Low/moderate severity: 7 days total.
  - High severity: 10–14 days total (not all IV).
  - Consider extending to 21 days total for *S. aureus* and Gram-negative bacilli.

Reference: British Thoracic Society Guidelines 2009.

Complications of pneumonia

- Pleural effusion:
  - Develops in 30–50% patients with CAP, often a cause of treatment failure.
  - All patients with parapneumonic effusion need thoracocentesis.
  - Complicated parapneumonic effusions (clear fluid with pH <7.2) need drainage.

- Empyema:
  - ◆ Pleural effusion with cloudy fluid, pus, organisms on Gram stain or culture.
  - ◆ Treatment: intercostal drain.
- Lung abscess:
  - ◆ More common in alcoholics and aspiration pneumonia.
  - ◆ Treatment: up to 6 weeks of antibiotics ± surgical drainage.
- Metastatic infection/septic emboli.

Bacterial infection

Streptococcus pneumoniae

- Most common pathogen cultured from blood or sputum.
- Features: increasing age, comorbidity, acute onset, pyrexia, pleuritic chest pain.
- Diagnosis: urinary antigen testing gives rapid diagnosis but no sensitivities.
- Treatment: amoxicillin/clarithromycin.
- Vaccination: recommended for asplenic patients, those with chronic cardiac, renal, or liver disease; give every 3 years.

Mycoplasma pneumoniae

- Peaks every 4 years.
- Features: younger patients, prior antibiotics, often preceding 'flu like illness:
  - ◆ Low platelets.
  - ◆ Rash: erythema multiforme or Stevens–Johnson syndrome.
  - ◆ Cold agglutinins cause autoimmune haemolytic anaemia.
  - ◆ SIADH.
  - ◆ Neurological complications: rarely Guillain–Barré syndrome/myelitis.
- Diagnosis: confirm with PCR or complement fixation test (CFT).
- Treatment: clarithromycin.

Legionella pneumophila

- >90% associated with foreign travel; outbreaks from air conditioning; peak incidence June–October in the UK.
- Features: young smokers, no comorbidity, more severe infection, deranged liver function tests (LFTs), raised creatine kinase (CK), hyponatraemia, neurological symptoms (confusion), and diarrhoea.
- Diagnosis: urinary antigen is sensitive and specific; culture and serology also available; culture must be sent if urinary antigen positive.
- A notifiable disease: inform the Health Protection Agency.
- Treatment: fluoroquinolones, e.g. ciprofloxacin.

Chlamydia psittaci (psittacosis)

- History of contact with birds in 10%.
- Features: prolonged symptoms and headache; hepatitis, rash, renal failure, rarely splenomegaly.
- Treatment: doxycycline.

Coxiella burnetii ('Q fever')

- Occasionally history of contact with sheep.
- Features: males > females, dry cough, and high fever.
- Diagnosis: PCR for BAL samples; otherwise CFT or direct immunofluorescence.
- Treatment: doxycycline.

Klebsiella pneumonia

- More common in males.
- Features: thrombocytopenia and leucopenia; high risk of sepsis and death in alcoholics.
- Treatment: IV cephalosporins.

Methicillin-resistant Staphylococcus aureus (MRSA)

- Genuine MRSA sepsis rare but high mortality (colonization common).
- Treatment: vancomycin or teicoplanin if sepsis suspected.

Panton-Valentine leukocidin producing Staphylococcus aureus (PVL-SA)

- Rare cause of severe pneumonia with cavitating disease.
- High mortality due to multiorgan failure.
- Treatment: clindamycin or linezolid plus rifampicin.

Viral infection

- Account for 13% of CAP (around 11% Influenza A and B).
- 10% of confirmed viral pneumonia complicated by co-infection with *S. aureus*.
- Influenza vaccination (A+B) recommended in:
  - At-risk groups: diabetes mellitus (DM), chronic asthma, COPD, renal, cardiac and other chronic disease, aged >65 years old.
  - Healthcare workers.

Severe acute respiratory syndrome (SARS)

- Outbreak in China 2002 plus occasional smaller outbreaks since.
- Coronavirus (SARS-CoV).
- Overall mortality 10%.

H1N1—swine 'flu

- H1N1 subtype of influenza A; originated in pigs but passed between humans.
- Typically presents as mild viral illness ± acute respiratory distress.
- More severe in young/pregnant patients.
- Management: oseltamivir (Tamiflu) or zanamivir (Relenza); best initiated within first 48 hrs; both safe in pregnancy.
- Vaccination: monovalent vaccine recommended for all at-risk groups.

H5N1—bird 'flu

- Endemic in some Eastern avian populations; human-to-human transmission rare.
- High human fatality rate (respiratory disease/adult respiratory distress syndrome (ARDS)).
- Treatment: oseltamivir may be of some benefit.
- Vaccination: rapid mutation of H5N1 makes available vaccines ineffective.

Cytomegalovirus (CMV) pneumonia

- A cause of pneumonia in immunocompromised patients, especially post bone marrow or solid organ transplant.
- Most cases seen within 4 months of transplant.
- CXR: hazy infiltrates or frank consolidation.
- Diagnosis: IgG positivity shows previous exposure not definite current infection; confirm with PCR or immunofluorescence testing of BAL or serum.
- Treatment: ganciclovir (causes anaemia, neutropenia) or foscarnet (renal toxicity).

Varicella pneumonia

- Occurs with either chicken pox or shingles.
- Higher risk if pregnant or immunocompromised.
- Rash plus cough, pleuritic chest pain, and haemoptysis.
- CXR: diffuse small nodules which can calcify and therefore persist for life.
- Concurrent bacterial infection common.
- Treatment: acyclovir ± antibiotics.

Measles pneumonia/pneumonitis

- Associated with pneumonia in adults.
- Previously rare but recent outbreaks following low immunization uptake.
- CXR: non-specific infiltrates, occasional consolidation.
- Treatment: supportive.

Fungal lung disease

Aspergillus

- Dichotomous branching ubiquitous fungus, *Aspergillus fumigatus* is most common pathogen.
- Allergic bronchopulmonary aspergillosis:
  - Normal/overactive immune system and allergic response to inhaled spores leading to asthma-like picture.
  - CXR: flitting infiltrates and proximal bronchiectasis.
  - Raised blood eosinophils, IgE (>1000 ng/ml), positive specific IgE to *Aspergillus* and positive *Aspergillus* precipitins (IgG) suggestive but not diagnostic.
  - Treatment: inhaled/oral steroids; trial of antifungal, e.g. itraconazole.
- Aspergilloma:
  - Relatively normal immune system but underlying lung disease, e.g. COPD, sarcoidosis, previous TB.
  - Fungus inhaled into pre-existing cavity and grows into fungal ball (mycetoma).
  - CXR/CT: cavity with fungal ball.
  - Treatment: prolonged course of itraconazole/fluconazole; resection if fit.
  - Complications: haemoptysis: treat with antibiotics, tranexamic acid ± arterial embolization (specialist centres only).
- Invasive/semi-invasive aspergillosis:
  - Severely immunocompromised host with invasion of fungus into tissue.
  - Entry via lungs but haematogenous spread to any organ (especially central nervous system (CNS), sinuses, skin, heart valves, and eyes); high mortality.

- ♦ CT: halo sign on CT.
- ♦ Treatment: parenteral antifungals, e.g. liposomal amphotericin.

Pneumocystis pneumonia (PCP)

- Fungus *Pneumocystis jiroveci*.
- Most common in HIV patients with CD4 <200; also post solid organ transplantation.
- Slow onset shortness of breath (SOB) and dry cough typical with oxygen desaturation on exercise.
- CXR: 10% normal, most commonly bilateral perihilar infiltrates and pneumothorax; effusions rare.
- Diagnosis: immunofluorescence on BAL/induced sputum.
- Prophylaxis: low-dose co-trimoxazole (Septrin) or pentamadine nebulizers.
- Treatment: high-dose (weight dependent) co-trimoxazole plus steroids if hypoxic.

Histoplasmosis/coccidiomycosis/paracoccidiomycosis

- Can all produce both asymptomatic and symptomatic infection.
- Symptomatic infection more common in immunocompromised patients.

Cryptococcus neoformans

- Inhaled spores (bird droppings) migrate from lungs causing meningoencephalitis.
- More common in immunocompromised patients.
- Chest signs unreliable.
- Diagnosis: CXR non-specific; BAL latex agglutination test or India Ink on cerebrospinal fluid (CSF); cryptococcal antigen test on serum or CSF highly specific and sensitive.
- Treatment: fluconazole for 6–12 months.

Candida spp.

- *Candida* commonly isolated from sputum but rarely pathological.
- Candidaemia more likely in severe neutropenia/post transplant or associated with parental feeding/central lines.
- 30–50% mortality.
- Diagnosis: positive culture from ≥2 sites.
- Treatment: amphotericin or fluconazole.

Parasitic lung disease

Localized infection

- Pulmonary hydatid:
  - ♦ Ingestion of eggs from faeces of animal carriers (dogs, sheep, cattle) in endemic areas.
  - ♦ *Echinococcus granulosus* larvae grow in the lungs causing cystic disease.
  - ♦ *Echinococcus multilocularis* causes more diffuse alveolar disease.
- Amoebic pulmonary disease:
  - ♦ Secondary infection with *Entamoeba histolytica* via blood or lymph from gastrointestinal (GI) tract or liver.
  - ♦ Abscesses, fistulae, or frank consolidation (and effusion) normally right sided.

- Filiariasis:
  - Worms in pulmonary arterial system cause distal infarct and often single inflammatory nodule.
  - Can be asymptomatic detectable on CXR.

Hypersensitivity reactions

- May manifest as any of wheeze, cough, rash, pleuritic chest pain, pulmonary infiltrates, and blood eosinophilia.
- Occurs with *Ascaris lumbricoides*, *Schiztosoma*, *Stongyloidydes stercoralis*, *Toxocara canis*, *Wuchereria bancrofti/Brugia malayi*.
- See Chapter 9: Eosinophilic lung disease.

Immunocompromised host

HIV positive patients

- Infection will depend on CD4 count.
- Most common pulmonary infection is bacterial pneumonia; pulmonary tuberculosis occurs regardless of CD4.
- Viral: *Cytomegalovirus*, varicella zoster, herpes simplex.
- Fungal: *Cryptococcus*, *Candida*, *Histoplasma*.
- CD4 <200: PCP and extrapulmonary tuberculosis.
- CD4 <50: non-tuberculous mycobacteria (*Mycobacterium avium-intracellulare, M. kansasii*), Kaposi's sarcoma (pleural or parenchymal), lymphoma.

HIV negative patients

- Impaired T-lymphocyte function, e.g. post transplant, lymphoma:
  - Bacterial: mycobacteria, *Leigonella*, *Listeria*, plus encapsulated bacteria (*Streptococcus* and *Haemophilus*) if B cells affected.
  - Fungal: PCP, *Cryptococcus*, *Candida*.
  - Parasitic infections.
- Impaired neutrophil function, e.g. post chemotherapy, leukaemia:
  - Bacterial: *Pseudomonas*, *Klebsiella*, *Staphylococcus*.
  - Fungal: *Aspergillus*, *Candida*.

Myobacterium tuberculosis (MTB)

Screening for MTB

- New UK entrants aged <35 years (age >35 years hepatoxicity risk exceeds benefit of treatment); NHS employees; opportunistic screening of homeless persons.

Reference: National Institute of Health and Clinical Excellence Guidelines 2006.

Latent tuberculosis (LTB)

- Risk factors:
  - Previous exposure to MTB with incomplete clearance ('dormant' disease).
  - Risk of reactivation higher in IV drug users, HIV positive, haematological malignancy, transplant, gastrectomy, dialysis, anti-TNF, silicosis.
- Diagnosis:
  - Tuberculin skin test (TST):
    - E.g. Mantoux (replaced Heaf testing in 2005).
    - False positive results with non-tuberculous mycobacteria (NTM) or Bacille Calmette–Guérin (BCG) vaccination.
    - False negative results with immunocompromise, steroid use, HIV, sarcoid, military TB (can be anergic—no response).
  - Interferon gamma release assay testing (IGRAs):
    - E.g. QuantiFERON-TB gold, T-SPOT.TB.
    - Used as the sole test for LTB in immune compromised individuals and in large-scale population screening.
    - Indicated to confirm a positive TST.
    - Not affected by BCG previous vaccination.
    - Not positive with most environmental mycobacteria.
  - If TST/IGRA positive, perform CXR to exclude active pulmonary TB.
- Indications for treatment:
  - ≤35 years old (or any age as healthcare worker).
  - Positive IGRA.
  - Positive Mantoux:
    - ≥15 mm with prior BCG vaccination.
    - ≥6 mm with no prior BCG vaccination.
  - CXR consistent with MTB (apical scars etc.) and no history of treatment.
  - No constitutional symptoms/signs suggestive of active disease.
- Treatment 'chemoprophylaxis':
  - 6 months of isoniazid or 3 months of rifinah (isoniazid and rifampicin).
  - HIV positive: 6 months of isoniazid.

Active tuberculosis

- Clinical features:
  - ◆ Cough, fever, weight loss, night sweats, often of several weeks' duration.
- Diagnosis:
  - ◆ Positive culture of MTB is the gold standard; takes up to 6 weeks.
  - ◆ TST and IGRAs not recommended as first-line investigations.
  - ◆ Pulmonary tuberculosis (PTB):
    - Take CXR; if this suggests PTB arrange further investigation.
    - Send ≥ 3 morning sputum samples for culture and microscopy.
    - Detection of acid-fast bacilli (AFB) on microscopy of ≥2 sputum smears (i.e. 'smear positive') is adequate for diagnosis.
  - ◆ Extrapulmonary tuberculosis (EPTB):
    - Send biopsy/fluid aspirate for culture and microscopy.
    - Detection of AFB on biopsy is adequate for diagnosis.
    - Perform a CXR for concurrent PTB.
- Pre-treatment screening:
  - ◆ U&E, LFT, FBC, vitamin D, HIV test.
  - ◆ Eye tests: colour vision (Ishihara chart) and acuity.
  - ◆ Assessment of probable compliance.
  - ◆ Assessment of risk of drug-resistant MTB.
  - ◆ Contact tracing.
  - ◆ Notify the HPA.
- Treatment:
  - ◆ Start treatment without culture results if there are signs and symptoms of MTB; complete the course even if culture results are negative.
- Quadruple therapy regimen:
  - ◆ Indicated for fully sensitive MTB at all sites except CNS.
  - ◆ Induction phase—2 months:
    - Rifampicin (R) isoniazid (H), ethambutol (E), pyrazinamide (Z).
    - Rifater (RHZ) plus ethambutol (E).
  - ◆ Consolidation phase—4 months:
    - Rifampicin and isoniazid.
  - ◆ Written as 2HRZE/4HR.
  - ◆ First choice should be to use fixed-dose tablets and daily dosing.

Special considerations

- Meningeal TB:
  - ◆ 12 months of treatment 2HRZE/10HE.
  - ◆ *Plus* glucocorticoid 20 mg (40 mg if on rifampicin).
- Bone TB:
  - ◆ Standard treatment.
  - ◆ Treat for meningeal TB if spinal cord involved.
  - ◆ Consider anterior spinal fusion for instability/compression.
- Miliary TB:
  - ◆ Standard treatment.
  - ◆ Treat for meningeal TB if CNS is involved.

- Pericardial TB:
  - Standard treatment.
  - *Plus* glucocorticoid 60 mg/day for 2 weeks then reduce.

Side effects of commonly used antituberculous drugs

- Rifampicin:
  - Hepatic enzyme inducer: reduces effectiveness of oral contraceptive pill; halves therapeutic level of prednisolone.
  - Hepatitis: tolerate alanine transaminase (ALT) to 5× baseline, stop if jaundiced.
  - Orange/red discoloration of all secretions.
- Isoniazid:
  - Age-dependent hepatitis.
  - Peripheral neuropathy: increased risk with pregnancy and diabetes; give pyridoxine (vitamin B1) to reduce risk.
  - Agranulocytosis.
- Pyrazinamide:
  - Hepatitis; gastrointestinal disturbance; arthralgia.
- Ethambutol:
  - Optic neuritis: colour vision affected first, often reversible.
- Streptomycin:
  - Oto/vestibular toxicity: tinnitus, vertigo, deafness.

Directly observed therapy (DOT)

- Treatment support with a named key worker; 3× per week supervised ingestion of antituberculous medication.
- Consider for patients with predicted poor adherence, concurrent alcohol or IV drug use, homelessness, or mental illness.

Drug resistance

- Simple drug resistance:
  - Resistance to 1 first-line agent, most commonly isoniazid.
- Multidrug resistance (MDR):
  - Resistance to ≥ 2 first-line agents including isoniazid and rifampicin.
- Extensively drug resistance (XDR):
  - Resistance to first- and second-line agents.
  - I.e. MDR TB with resistance to any fluoroquinolone and at least 1 of the IV agents kanamycin, capreomycin, and amikacin.
- Risk factors for resistance:
  - Prior TB treatment or treatment failure.
  - Contact of known case of resistant TB.
  - Birth in a country with high rates of resistance or residence in London.
  - HIV infection.
- Perform rapid molecular testing on all suspected cases.
- Consider compulsory medical examination/hospital admission under the Public Health Act 1984 and Health Protection Regulations 2010.
- Treat MDR with at least 3 agents and XDR with at least 5 agents to which the organism is likely to be sensitive.

- Review regimen if cultures remain positive after 4 months.
- Extend treatment course up to 2 years with 12 months' follow-up post treatment.

Screening pre anti-TNF therapy

- Screen all patients before starting anti-TNF therapy with history/CXR:
  - Normal CXR not on immunosuppressants: TST.
  - Normal CXR on immunosuppressants: IGRA and risk stratification.
- If CXR abnormal with history of fully treated TB:
  - Monitor.
- If CXR abnormal with history of inadequately treated TB:
  - Complete chemoprophylaxis (3 months of rifinah or 6 months of isoniazid) before starting anti-TNF.
- If evidence of active TB:
  - Complete 6 months of standard treatment; minimum 2 months of treatment before starting anti-TNF.

Reference: British Thoracic Society Guidelines 2005.

Chronic kidney disease and TB

- Risk of developing active TB is 20× greater in patients with CKD; often EPTB.
- Consider screening for LTB pre-transplant:
  - CXR + IGRA ± TST (TST only helpful if positive).
  - Offer treatment for LTB if abnormal CXR and/or positive IGRA/TST.

Reference: British Thoracic Society Guidelines 2010.

HIV and TB coinfection

- HIV is associated with an increased risk of activation of LTB, EPTB, miliary TB, and drug-resistant TB.
- Start TB therapy prior to HAART, otherwise immune reconstitution inflammatory syndrome (IRIS) may exacerbate TB:
  - Steroids may be used to dampen immune response.
  - CD4 <100 cells/µL: start HAART as soon as practical after TB therapy.
  - CD4 100–350 cells/µL: start HAART after 2 months of TB therapy.
  - CD4 consistently >350 cells/µL: start HAART at physician's discretion.
- Rifampicin induces CYP450 and interacts with protease inhibitors, NNRTIs, and antimicrobials such as fluconazole. Rifabutin is an alternative to rifampicin.

Reference: British HIV Association Guidelines 2010.

Vaccination

- Live attenuated strain of M. bovis; stimulates cross-immunity to M. tuberculosis and M. leprae.
- Most efficacious in preventing childhood TB meningitis (70–80% efficacy).
- Protective effect thought to last around 10 years.
- Indicated in:
  - neonates: born in a high-risk area or to parents/grandparents from a high-risk area or with a positive family history in the preceding 5 years
  - infants: 4 weeks to 16 years at increased risk and Mantoux negative

  ◆ new entrants to the UK: from a high-risk area with no previous vaccination *and* aged <16 *or* aged 16–35 years from sub-Saharan Africa
  ◆ healthcare workers: no previous vaccination, due patient contact, *and* Mantoux/IGRA negative
  ◆ contacts of patients with active TB: no previous vaccination, aged <35 years, *and* Mantoux negative.
- Contraindicated in HIV and pregnancy.

Non-tuberculous mycobacteria (NTM)

- Over 100 species—defined as slow growing and fast growing.
- Acquired from environmental exposure: no evidence of animal-to-human or human-to-human transmission.
- Asymptomatic colonization and pathological disease difficult to distinguish.
- Pathological disease affects lungs, lymphatics, and skin/soft tissue; disseminated disease also occurs.

Reference: British Thoracic Society Guidelines 2009.

Pulmonary disease

Slow growing mycobacteria

- *M. kansasii*, *M. avium* complex (MAC), *M. malmoense*, *M. xenopi*.
- Predisposing factors:
  ◆ Middle aged/elderly men.
  ◆ Structural lung disorders (COPD, bronchiectasis, CF, pneumoconiosis, prior TB, pulmonary alveolar proteinosis).
  ◆ Oesophageal motility disorders.
- Features:
  ◆ Variable and non-specific; chronic or recurring cough, sputum production, fatigue, malaise, dyspnoea, fever, haemoptysis, lethargy, and weight loss.
- Diagnosis:
  ◆ Consistent history and radiological findings:
    ▪ CXR: nodular or cavitary opacities (70–90%); often indistinguishable from MTB.
    ▪ HRCT: multifocal bronchiectasis.
  ◆ *Plus* ≥2 positive cultures from non-sterile sites (sputum) *or* single culture *or* consistent histopathology from sterile site (pleural fluid/lung biopsy).
- Treatment: 24 months of rifampicin and ethambutol (9 months for *M. kansasii*).
- No need to contact trace or notify.

Lady Windermere syndrome

- MAC pulmonary infection, limited to the right middle lobe or lingula, with localized bronchiectasis.
- Most commonly affects immunocompetent elderly women with no significant smoking history or underlying lung disease.
- May be related to voluntary cough suppression with failure to clear secretions.

Fast growing mycobacteria

- *M. chelonae, M. fortuitum, M. abscessus, M. gordonae.*
- Features:
  - Rare and difficult to treat.
- Treatment:
  - Combination of rifampicin, ethambutol and clarithromycin ± surgical resection; may not achieve cure.

HIV-positive patients

MAC

- Most common cause of disseminated NTM in HIV/AIDS.
- Frequency increases with falling CD4 count (CD4 <50).
- IRIS response may occur within 2 months of starting HAART.
- Rarely limited to the lungs; disseminated disease more common.
- Diagnosis:
  - Blood cultures positive in 95% with disseminated disease.
  - CXR: infiltrates, nodular disease, cavities rare.
- Prophylaxis:
  - Azithromycin lifelong.
- Treatment:
  - Rifampicin, ethambutol, and clarithro/azithromycin lifelong.

M. kansasii

- Second most common cause of disseminated NTM in HIV/AIDS.
- 50% confined to pulmonary disease.
- Often fatal.
- Treatment:
  - Rifampicin, ethambutol, clarithromycin ± isoniazid lifelong.

Bronchiectasis

Causes of bronchiectasis

- Idiopathic (approximately 50%).
- Post-infective:
  - ◆ *Klebsiella*, *S. aureus*, *Mycoplasma*, MTB, non-tuberculous mycobacterium (NTM) including MAC, viral respiratory infection.
- Bronchial obstruction.
- Aspiration.
- Cystic fibrosis (CF).
- Disorders of ciliary function:
  - ◆ Primary ciliary dyskinesia, Kartagener's syndrome, Young's syndrome.
- Immunodeficiency states:
  - ◆ Most commonly B lymphocyte disorders, e.g. common variable immunodeficiency, Ig subclass deficiency, X-linked agammaglobulinaemia.
- Congenital anatomic defects:
  - ◆ Williams Campbell syndrome: bronchial cartilage deficiency.
  - ◆ Mounier–Kuhn syndrome: tracheobronchomegaly.
  - ◆ Yellow nail syndrome: pleural effusions, nail dystrophy, sinusitis, lymphoedema.
- Autoimmune and connective-tissue disorders:
  - ◆ Rheumatoid arthritis, Sjögren's syndrome, inflammatory bowel disease (ulcerative colitis).
  - ◆ Marfan's syndrome: tracheobronchial and oesophagobronchial fistulae.
- A1AT deficiency, COPD, asthma, allergic bronchopulmonary aspergillosis (ABPA).
- Traction from other processes.

Investigations indicated in all patients

- Serum immunoglobulin levels (IgG, IgA, IgM) and serum electrophoresis.
- Immune function screening—assessment of humoral response:
  - ◆ Measure baseline tetanus and *Streptococcus* antibody levels, immunize and repeat levels at 21 days.
- Aspergillus:
  - ◆ Total IgE, IgE specific to *Aspergillus* (RAST), *Aspergillus* precipitins (IgG).
- Sputum microscopy and culture: persistent *S. aureus* suggests CF/ABPA.
- CXR: normal in ≈10%; repeat only if clinically indicated; HRCT if CXR inconclusive.
- PFTs: minimum FEV_1, FVC, and PEFR; obstructive pattern most common.

Investigations indicated in specific patients

- Ciliary function: saccharin test, exhaled nasal NO, cilial electron microscopy:
  - Indication: chronic upper respiratory tract problems/otitis media.
- Bronchoscopy:
  - Indication: localized disease to exclude proximal obstruction; HRCT suggestive of NTM infection with negative sputum culture.
- Screening for CF: sweat chloride ×2 plus genetic studies:
  - Indication: age <40 years or age >40 years with a suggestive history (persistent S. aureus positive sputum, childhood steatorrhoea, malabsorption, primary male infertility, upper lobe bronchiectasis).

Reference: British Thoracic Society Guidelines 2010

Radiological findings

- HRCT:
  - Bronchial wall dilation ± thickening.
  - Lack of tapering of the distal bronchus.
  - Internal diameter of bronchus > accompanying artery ('Signet ring' sign).
- Specific patterns of disease:
  - Localized disease: inhaled foreign body, proximal obstruction.
  - Upper lobe predominance: CF.
  - Upper lobe and central bronchiectasis: ABPA.
  - Upper lobe and tracheobrochomegaly with 'grape-like' bronchiectasis: Mounier–Kuhn syndrome.
  - Middle lobe and lingula with nodules and tree in bud opacification: Lady Windermere syndrome due to MAC.
  - Lower lobe predominance: ciliary dysfunction; chronic aspiration; A1AT deficiency.

Management

- Aim to reduce severity and frequency of exacerbations to slow disease progression.
- Identify and treat underlying cause.
- Mucus volume reduction and clearance: airway clearance techniques, bronchodilators, saline or hypertonic saline nebulizers, mucolytics (avoid recombinant human deoxyribonuclease (rhDNAse) unless CF).
- Sputum surveillance and prompt treatment of infective exacerbations:
  - Colonization: H. influenzae > Pseudomonas > S. pneumoniae
  - Isolation of a new strain of H. influenzae, M. catarrhalis, or S. pneumoniae is associated with an increased risk of exacerbation.
- Surgery and transplantation: resection for localized disease and uncontrolled haemoptysis, transplant for end-stage disease with respiratory failure.
- Pulmonary rehabilitation/inspiratory muscle training.
- Send sputum culture before initiating antibiotics.
- Empirical antibiotics:
  - 14 days of monotherapy with amoxicillin or clarithromycin.
  - Ciprofloxacin for patients colonized with Pseudomonas.
- Dual therapy for resistant Pseudomonas, MRSA, or recurrent infections.

- Long-term antibiotics for patients with ≥3 exacerbations per year:
  - Antibiotics guided by microbiology.
  - Nebulized colomycin/tobramycin if *Pseudomonas* colonization.
  - Possible disease-modifying action of azithromycin.
- Rotating antibiotics: used but with little evidence.

Reference: British Thoracic Society Guidelines 2010 Antibiotic guidance

Complications

- Recurrent infection, lung abscess, empyema, septic emboli.
- Haemoptysis: mild chronic haemoptysis from inflamed airways or massive haemoptysis (>250 ml/24 hrs) from tortuous dilated bronchial vessels.
- Broncho-pleural fistulae and pneumothoraces.
- Right heart failure/cor pulmonale.
- Respiratory failure.
- Amyloidosis.

Cystic fibrosis

- Autosomal recessive; 1:25 carrier frequency and 1:2500 live births in Caucasians.
- Mutation of cystic fibrosis transmembrane regulator (*CFTR*) gene:
  - Long arm of chromosome 7; >1500 mutations recognized.
  - In UK around 70% due to deletion of phenylalanine at codon 508 (ΔF508).
- Epithelial cell chloride channel defect causes increased cell sodium uptake and increased viscosity of secretions.

Diagnosis

- Newborn screening: heel prick 'Guthrie test'—immunoreactive trypsin.
- Sweat testing: Cl^- >60 mmol/L is diagnostic.
- *CFTR* genetic studies.
- Supportive tests: nasal potential difference; faecal elastase.

Annual surveillance

- PFTs including plethysmography, lung clearance index (sulphur hexafluoride), CXR, USS liver and spleen, dual-emission X-ray absorptiometry (DEXA), oral glucose tolerance test (OGTT), sputum microscopy and culture including NTM, bloods (FBC, U&Es, LFTs, bone profile, vitamins A, D, & E, iron studies, immunoglobulin profile, *Aspergillus* profile), nutritional assessment.
- Segregate clinic patients with *Burkholderia cepacia*, MRSA, mucoid/multiresistant *Pseudomonas*, respiratory viruses.

Common pathogens

- Early: transition from sterile airways with transient infection with *H. influenza*, *S. aureus*, and *Pseudomonas* to chronic colonization with these organisms:
  - Mucoid phenotype of *P. aeruginosa* predominates (biofilm producing).
- Late: infection ± colonization with *Burkholderia cepacia*, *Stenotrophomonas maltophila*, *Alccaligenes xylosoxidans*, opportunistic NTM, *Candida*, and *Aspergillus*.

Complications and management

Respiratory

- Infective exacerbation:
  - ◆ Prophylaxis: antibiotic therapy, e.g. flucloxacillin (*S. aureus*).
  - ◆ Rapid specific treatment for infective exacerbations.
  - ◆ Long-term antibiotics—reduce bacterial load:
    - ▪ ≥2 isolates/year *S. aureus* (flucloxacillin/augmentin) or *H. influenzae* (augmentin).
    - ▪ Recurrent *Pseudomonas*: nebulized colistin/tobramycin.
  - ◆ Anti-inflammatory/immune modulation: azithromycin.
  - ◆ ± Portacath: risk of occlusion, infection, fracture, embolization.
  - ◆ Airway clearance techniques:
    - ▪ Active cycle breathing, PEEP, flutter, acapella.
    - ▪ Bronchodilators, hypertonic saline, rhDNAse.
- *Aspergillus* lung disease:
  - ◆ ABPA: itraconazole plus steroids (oral/IV).
  - ◆ Invasive aspergillosis: IV liposomal amphotericin (ambisome).
  - ◆ Aspergilloma: surgical resection.
- Pneumothorax:
  - ◆ Incidence increases with age and disease severity.
  - ◆ Localized abrasion pleurodesis/stapling of blebs recommended.
  - ◆ Avoid talc pleurodesis and total pleurectomy (detrimental to transplant).
- Haemoptysis:
  - ◆ Massive haemoptysis affects 1% per year.
  - ◆ Lie on affected side.
  - ◆ Give supplementary oxygen, tranexamic acid, and IV antibiotics to cover *S. aureus*.
  - ◆ Transfuse and correct coagulopathy.
  - ◆ ± IV terlipressin, bronchoscopy and bronchial angiography/embolization:
    - ▪ Often multiple vessels involved; risk of spinal artery occlusion.
  - ◆ ± Intubate with double lumen tube and ventilate good lung.
  - ◆ Emergency surgical resection (high risk) if embolization fails.
- Respiratory failure:
  - ◆ LTOT for hypoxia.
  - ◆ NIV for type II respiratory failure and as a bridge to transplant.
  - ◆ Transplantation most commonly double lung; previously domino.

Reference: Royal Brompton Hospital Guidelines 2011.

Non-respiratory

- ENT complications:
  - ◆ Nasal polyposis affects up to 50% of adults with CF.
  - ◆ Chronic sinusitis is almost universal.
- Gastrointestinal complications:
  - ◆ Pancreatic insufficiency: pancrealipase (Creon) supplements pre-meal.
  - ◆ Hepatobiliary complications: involve hepatologist early:
    - ▪ Steatosis (fatty liver) affects up to 70%.
    - ▪ Gallstones, cholecyctitis, biliary cirrhosis, portal hypertension.
    - ▪ Treat with ursodeoxycholic acid ± vitamin K; prophylaxis *not* recommended.

- ◆ Distal intestinal obstructive syndrome (DIOS): accumulation of viscid faecal material; treat acute episodes with oral gastrograffin.
- CF-related diabetes (CFRD):
  - ◆ Insulin deficiency associated with pancreatic insufficiency.
  - ◆ Insulin therapy reduces the detrimental effect of CFRD on life expectancy.
  - ◆ Oral agents *not* recommended.
- Growth and puberty:
  - ◆ Calorific requirements 50% higher than healthy individuals.
  - ◆ High-fat, high-energy diet recommended.
  - ◆ May require nasogastric/gastrostomy feeding:
    - ± Elemental feed with medium chain triglycerides as fat source.
  - ◆ Puberty often delayed; affects bone density; treat with sex steroids.
- Bone metabolism:
  - ◆ Osteopaenia/porosis affects up to 33% of adults with CF.
  - ◆ Arthropathy affects up to 10%: usually large joints.
  - ◆ Minimize steroid use; ensure adequate oral calcium intake.
  - ◆ Maintain serum 25 hydroxy vitamin D >75 nmol/L:
    - 400 IU vitamin D daily prophylaxis (with vitamin A/multivitamins).
    - Additional supplementation if level <50 nmol/L.
  - ◆ Bisphosphonates indicated only if fractures occur.
- Fertility:
  - ◆ Around 98% of male patients are infertile (although not sterile) due to congenital absence of vas deferens; assisted conception possible.
  - ◆ Female patients have cervical mucus thickening and impaired sperm transfer but can usually conceive naturally.
  - ◆ Beware of progesterone-only contraception which can reduce bone density.
- Psychological/psychiatric complications.

Reference: Royal Brompton Hospital Guidelines 2011.

INTERSTITIAL LUNG DISEASE

Classification of interstitial lung disease (ILD)

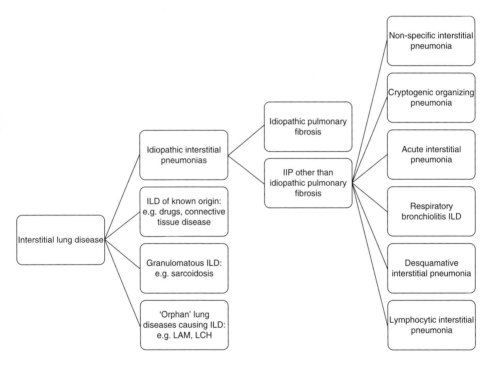

Idiopathic interstitial pneumonia (IIP)

Diagnosis

- History, examination, and compatible radiology (CXR/HRCT) may be sufficient for diagnosis; if not, BAL ± transbronchial lung biopsy (TBLB) may be required.
- Laboratory investigations:
  - FBC, U&Es, LFTs, urine dipstick.
  - ± Rheumatoid factor, antinuclear antibodies, extractable nuclear antigens, IgG precipitins, serum angiotensin-converting enzyme (ACE), depending on clinical context.
- Radiology:
  - Sensitivity of CXR for ILD is 80%; sensitivity of HRCT for ILD is 94%.

- ◆ HCRT changes:
  - Ground glass: inflammatory process, often steroid responsive.
  - Reticulation/honeycombing: non-reversible fibrotic process.
- BAL:
  - ◆ More useful in the diagnosis of opportunistic infection, malignancy, acute eosinophilic pneumonia, and alveolar proteinosis than the common ILDs.
  - ◆ Indicated in all patients undergoing TBLB.
  - ◆ Risks: as per bronchoscopy—major complication rate <0.5%, mortality <0.05%.
- TBLB:
  - ◆ Indicated when small histological samples may be diagnostic; especially bronchocentric disease, e.g. sarcoidosis, malignancy, COP:
    - Surgical lung biopsy is preferable in IPF.
  - ◆ 4–6 transbronchial samples should be taken:
    - Plus endobronchial samples in suspected sarcoidosis.
  - ◆ Risks: pneumothorax 1–2%, significant haemorrhage 1–4%, mortality 0.1%.
- Surgical lung biopsy:
  - ◆ Used to confirm pathological diagnosis.
  - ◆ More than one biopsy sample is required from more than one lobe:
    - Biopsy sites guided by HRCT findings.
  - ◆ VATs is preferable to open lung biopsy.
  - ◆ Risks: complication rate 7% (mostly pain/persistent air leak), mortality 1%.

Disease-specific features: in order of descending disease frequency

- Idiopathic pulmonary fibrosis (IPF):
  - ◆ HRCT: bibasal, peripheral, subpleural reticulation, minimal ground glass.
  - ◆ BAL: typically raised neutrophils (>4%) and eosinophils (>2%).
  - ◆ Histology: (described as usual interstitial pneumonia (UIP)) scattered areas of fibroblastic foci and honeycombing reflecting the spatial and temporal heterogeneity of fibrosis, minimal inflammation.
- Non-specific interstitial pneumonia (NSIP):
  - ◆ HRCT: bilateral, diffuse ground glass change, confluent and symmetrical, reticulation rare.
  - ◆ BAL: typically raised granulocytes.
  - ◆ Histology: spectrum from predominantly interstitial inflammation to fibrosis; fibroblastic foci and honeycombing rarely seen.
- Cryptogenic organizing pneumonia (COP):
  - ◆ HRCT: consolidation with air bronchograms, basal, subpleural, and peribronchial; ground glass and nodules may be present; rarely presents as a single mass ± cavitation.
  - ◆ Histology: patchy plugging of the alveolar spaces with inflammatory products (inflammatory cells, fibroblasts, fibrin).
- Acute interstitial pneumonia (AIP):
  - ◆ HRCT: early—bilateral, diffuse ground glass change; late—reticulation, traction bronchiectasis and cystic change.
  - ◆ Histology: diffuse alveolar insult with interstitial inflammation, oedema, hyaline membrane formation, and septal thickening. Later there may be organizing fibrosis and honeycombing.
- Respiratory bronchiolitis-interstitial lung disease (RB-ILD):
  - ◆ HRCT: fine nodules, ground glass change, airway thickening; commonly associated with centrilobular emphysema.

- Histology: patchy accumulation of pigmented alveolar macrophages within terminal bronchioles.
- Desquamative interstitial pneumonia (DIP):
  - HRCT: basal, peripheral ground glass change ± mild reticulation.
  - Histology: diffuse, uniform accumulation of pigmented macrophages within alveolar air space.
- Lymphocytic interstitial pneumonia (LIP):
  - HRCT: basal ground glass change ± nodules and reticulation.
  - Histology: diffuse interstitial lymphoid infiltrates involving alveolar septa.

Risk factors

- Smoking:
  - An independent risk factor for IPF (odds ratio 1.6–2.9).
  - RB-ILD, DIP, and Langerhans cell histiocytosis (LCH) occur almost exclusively in smokers.
  - Smokers are less likely to have hypersensitivity pneumonitis or sarcoidosis.

Assessment of severity

- Severity is best staged by TLCO (IPF/NSIP):
  - TLCO >40%: limited disease, extended survival more likely.
  - TLCO <40%: advanced disease.
- FVC on serial lung function testing most consistently predicts mortality (IPF):
  - Decrease in FVC ≥10% from baseline.
  - Or decrease in TLCO ≥15% in the first 6–12 months.
- Desaturation on 6MWT is a stronger indicator of prognosis than resting PFTs (IPF).

Management

- Refer to a MDT, based in a regional centre, with expertise in ILD.
- General/supportive measures:
  - Smoking cessation.
  - Pulmonary rehabilitation.
  - Oxygen therapy:
    - LTOT for PaO_2 ≤7.3 kPa or <8 kPa with pulmonary hypertension.
    - Ambulatory oxygen if symptoms of dyspnoea or hypoxia on exertion.
  - Proton pump inhibitors for all symptomatic patients.
  - Consider referral for transplant assessment in advanced/progressive disease.
  - Early recognition of terminal decline and palliative care.
- Disease specific:
  - IPF:
    - No therapy proven to modify clinical course or improve outcome.
    - Combination therapy historically recommended:
      - Prednisolone (tapering from 0.5 mg/kg to 10–20 mg/day).
      - Azathioprine (2 mg/kg, max. 150 mg/day).
      - N-acetyl-cysteine (600 mg three times a day).
    - Current evidence suggests triple therapy may be detrimental:
      - Avoid commencing triple therapy.
      - Cease azathioprine if there is disease progression.
    - Avoid steroid monotherapy.

♦ Connective tissue disease-associated ILD:
  ▪ Avoid high-dose steroids in systemic sclerosis—risk of renal crisis.
    ▸ Prednisolone (tapering from 0.5–1.0 mg/kg to ≤10 mg/day).
    ▸ ± Immunosuppressants (azathioprine/ cyclophosphamide).

Reference: British Thoracic Society Guidelines 2008.

Complications

- Spontaneous pneumothorax/pneumomediastinum.
- Pulmonary hypertension/cor pulmonale.
- Increased risk of small cell and non-small cell cancer, independent of smoking history.

Other lung diseases causing ILD

Drug induced

- E.g. Busulphan, bleomycin, gold, sulphasalazine, methotrexate, cyclophosphamide, nitrofurantoin, amiodarone.

Hypersensitivity pneumonitis

- Reaction to inhalation of antigen for which sensitization has previously occurred.
- Type III (cell mediated) or type IV (immune complex) reaction.
- Not an atopic condition; no eosinophilic response.
- Antigens:
  ♦ Farmer's lung: mouldy hay—*Thermophilic actinomycetes*, *Aspergillus*, *Micropolyspora faeni*.
  ♦ Bagassosis: mouldy sugarcane—*Thermophilic actinomycetes*.
  ♦ Bird fancier's lung: bird droppings and feathers—avian precipitins.
  ♦ Malt worker's lung: mouldy barley—*Aspergillus clavatus*.
  ♦ Hot tub lung: *Mycobacterium avium* complex.
  ♦ Isocyanate hypersensitivity: paints/resins/polyurethane.
- Presentation:
  ♦ Acute: flu-like illness.
  ♦ Subacute: recurrent pneumonia type symptoms.
  ♦ Chronic: cough, progressive dyspnoea, fatigue, weight loss.
- Peribronchial, non-caseating granulomata appear micronodular on CXR.
- Persistent antigen insult leads to progressive fibrosis of the upper lobes.
- BAL: lymphocytosis >40%; serum: neutrophilia.
- Pulmonary function tests: restrictive with reduced lung volumes and TLCO.
- Management:
  ♦ Allergen avoidance; full recovery common if exposure terminated early.
  ♦ ± Corticosteroids (poor evidence).

Granulomatous disease: sarcoidosis

- Symptoms:
  ♦ 5% are asymptomatic and detected incidentally by CXR.
  ♦ Cough, exertional dyspnoea, chest pain, fever, anorexia, arthralgia.
- Löfgren's syndrome:
  ♦ Fever, hilar lymphadenopathy, and polyarthralgias.

- ◆ Resolves spontaneously in 80% over 2 years.
- Extrapulmonary disease:
  - ◆ Dermatological: erythema nodosum, lupus pernio.
  - ◆ Ophthalmological: uveitis, episcleritis, scleritis, glaucoma, conjunctivitis, retinal involvement, keratoconjunctivitis sicca.
  - ◆ Cardiac: cardiomyopathy, conduction defects, sudden cardiac death.
  - ◆ Neurological: cranial nerve palsies, lymphocytic meningitis.
- Diagnosis:
  - ◆ Requires compatible clinical, radiological, and histological findings; without these, sarcoidosis is a diagnosis of exclusion:
    - ■ Löfgren's syndrome can be diagnosed without a biopsy.
  - ◆ Haematology: lymphopenia during the acute phase, serum ACE elevated in 60% at diagnosis (sensitivity 60%, specificity 70%), baseline LFTs, serum and urine calcium.
  - ◆ ECG for ST segment abnormalities and conduction block.
  - ◆ BAL typically lymphocytic.
  - ◆ TBLB and endobronchial biopsy for non-caseating, epithelioid-cell granulomata:
    - ■ Diagnostic yield: TBLB up to 90%; endobronchial 41–77%.
    - ■ Combination increases diagnostic yield by 21%.
  - ◆ ± EBUS TBNA; sensitivity approximately 85%.
- Radiological classification:
  - ◆ I: hilar lymphadenopathy.
  - ◆ II: hilar lymphadenopathy and pulmonary infiltrates.
  - ◆ III: pulmonary infiltrates alone.
  - ◆ IV: pulmonary fibrosis.
- Management:
  - ◆ Not indicated in asymptomatic stage I, II, or III disease provided lung function is only mildly abnormal and not deteriorating.
  - ◆ Oral steroids indicated if progressive disease, significant symptoms or extrapulmonary disease:
    - ■ Prednisolone 0.5 mg/kg/day for 4 weeks.
    - ■ Maintenance dose for 6–24 months.
  - ◆ Vital capacity may be used to measure steroid responsiveness.
  - ◆ Bisphosphonates for osteoporosis prophylaxis.
  - ◆ Transplantation should be considered in end-stage disease.
- Prognosis:
  - ◆ Worse if age >40 years, Afro-carribean origin, stage III/IV disease.

Langerhans cell histiocytosis (LCH)

- Occurs almost exclusively in smokers; cigarette smoke induces recruitment of Langerhans cells to the lung.
- Proliferation of Langerhans cells occurs along small airways with nodule formation (1–5 mm diameter), cystic change, and fibrosis.
- Predominantly middle/upper lobe disease, sparing the costophrenic angles.
- Histology: CD1 antigen positivity; Birbeck granules on electron microscopy.
- PFTs: obstructive/restrictive/mixed with reduced DLCO.
- Management:
  - ◆ Smoking cessation.

◆ Corticosteroids (poor evidence).
◆ Transplantation.

Lymphangioleiomyomatosis (LAM)

- Sporadic form affects women of childbearing age.
- Hormone dependent, abnormal proliferation of smooth muscle growth in the airways, blood vessels, and lymphatics.
- Small airway obstruction, cystic change, recurrent pneumothoraces and lymphatic obstruction with chylous effusions/ascites.
- Pulmonary venule obstruction causes vascular congestion and haemoptysis.
- Management:
  ◆ No proven treatment exists—management is symptomatic.
  ◆ Smoking cessation.
  ◆ Avoid pregnancy and exogenous oestrogens.
  ◆ Transplantation for advanced disease.

Alveolar proteinosis

- Congenital, acquired, or secondary (silicosis, immunodeficiency disorders, e.g. thymic hypoplasia and IgA deficiency, haematological malignancy).
- Antibodies to granulocyte-macrophage colony-stimulating factor (GM-CSF) lead to impaired alveolar macrophage function.
- Intra-alveolar accumulation of lipoproteinaceous material (surfactant components/cellular debris) with minimal interstitial inflammation or fibrosis.
- PFTs: restrictive with reduced lung volumes and TLCO.
- Management:
  ◆ Supportive with whole lung lavage.
  ◆ Transplantation for advanced disease.
  ◆ Limited evidence for subcutaneous GM-CSF.

PULMONARY VASCULAR DISEASE

Pulmonary embolism (PE)

Risk factors

- Major (relative risk 5–20): recent surgery (abdominal/orthopaedic), postoperative ITU, late pregnancy/puerperium, Caesarean section, lower limb fracture, varicose veins, malignancy (abdominal/pelvic/metastatic), previous thromboembolism, immobility.
- Minor (relative risk 2–4): congenital heart disease, cardiac failure, hypertension, oestrogen supplementation, neurological disability, occult malignancy, thrombotic disorders, long distance travel, raised BMI.

Clinical findings (in order of decreasing prevalence)

- Symptoms: dyspnoea, pleuritic pain, subcostal pain, cough, haemoptysis, syncope.
- Signs: tachypnoea (≥20/min), tachycardia (>100/min), clinical deep vein thrombosis (DVT), fever (>38.5°C), cyanosis.

Investigation

- Assess probability of PE using a clinical scoring system, e.g. Wells score, Geneva score (see Chapter 16: Respiratory scoring systems and statistics).
- D-dimer:
  - Perform only if low or intermediate clinical probability of PE:
    - If negative, PE is reliably excluded.
  - False positives with sepsis, neoplasia, inflammation, trauma, pregnancy, etc.
- Imaging:
  - CT pulmonary angiogram (CTPA) recommended for initial imaging; if negative, PE is reliably excluded.
  - Isotope lung scanning may be used for initial imaging if:
    - facilities are available on site, CXR is normal, there is no concurrent cardiopulmonary disease, standardized reporting criteria are used, a non-diagnostic result is always followed by further imaging
    - if negative, PE is reliably excluded.
  - ECHO will confirm right ventricular (RV) strain/failure.
- The BTS recommend screening for thrombophilia (present in 25–50% with DVT/PE) in those aged <50 years with recurrent PE, or those with a strong family history.
- Investigations for occult cancer are only indicated if there is a clinical suspicion.

Reference: British Thoracic Society Guidelines 2003.

Poor prognostic indicators

- Haemodynamic compromise: shock, hypotension (systolic blood pressure <90 mmHg or sustained drop in systolic blood pressure ≥40 mmHg).
- RV dysfunction: RV dilatation, hypokinesis or pressure overload on cardiac imaging, raised brain natriuretic peptide (BNP), raised right heart pressures at cardiac catheterization.
- Myocardial injury: positive troponin.
- Mortality exceeds 15% for patients with haemodynamic compromise, RV dysfunction and myocardial injury:
  - ◆ In patients with none of these features, mortality is <1%.

Treatment

- First line:
  - ◆ Give heparin to patients with intermediate or high probability of PE.
  - ◆ Low-molecular-weight heparin is preferred to unfractionated heparin except in haemodynamic compromise or where rapid reversal may be needed.
  - ◆ Thrombolysis is first-line treatment if there is haemodynamic compromise: Alteplase 50 mg bolus IV.
  - ◆ Inferior vena cava filters may be used if anticoagulation is contraindicated or unsuccessful in preventing recurrent PE.
- Ongoing:
  - ◆ Oral anticoagulation:
    - Target international normalized ratio (INR) should be 2.0–3.0; once reached, stop heparin.
    - Duration: 4–6 weeks for temporary risk factors, 3 months for first idiopathic, and *at least* 6 months for other situations.
- Increase target INR to 3.5 if recurrent emboli on warfarin.

Reference: British Thoracic Society, 2003/ British Committee for Standards in Haematology Guidelines 2011.

Pregnancy

- In suspected acute PE, CXR should be performed; if this is normal, perform compression Doppler of the lower limbs. If Doppler is also negative, perform isotope scan or CTPA.
- Isotope scanning carries a greater risk of childhood cancer than CTPA (1:280,000 versus <1:1,000,000) but a lower risk of maternal breast cancer.
- In proven PE, treat with low-molecular-weight heparin until at least 6 weeks post delivery, for a total of not less than 3 months.

Reference : Royal College of Obstetricians and Gynaecologists Guidelines 2007.

Pulmonary hypertension

Definition

- Pulmonary hypertension: mean pulmonary arterial pressure (mPAP) ≥25 mmHg at rest or ≥30 mmHg on exertion.
- Pulmonary arterial hypertension: mPAP ≥25 mmHg plus PCWP/LAP ≤15 mmHg plus PVR >3 Woods units.

Classification

- 1: Pulmonary arterial hypertension (PAH):
  - Idiopathic.
  - Familial: defects in BMPR2/ALK 1.
  - Drug/toxin induced: e.g. fenfluramine, dexfenfluramine, toxic rapeseed oil, amphetamines, L-tryptophan.
  - Associated with: connective tissue disease, HIV infection, portal hypertension, congenital heart disease, chronic haemolytic anaemia.
  - Persistent pulmonary hypertension of the newborn.
- 1': Pulmonary veno-occlusive disease and/or pulmonary capillary haemangiomatosis.
- 2: Pulmonary hypertension due to left heart disease.
- 3: Pulmonary hypertension due to lung disease and/or hypoxia.
- 4: Chronic thromboembolic pulmonary hypertension.
- 5: Miscellaneous:
  - Haematological: myeloproliferative disorders, splenectomy.
  - Systemic: sarcoidosis, LCH, LAM, neurofibromatosis, vasculitis.
  - Metabolic: glycogen storage disorders, Gaucher's, thyroid disease.
  - Other: tumour obstruction, fibrosing mediastinitis, dialysis.

Reference : European Society of Cardiology/ European Respiratory Society Guidelines 2009.

Investigation

- Haematology:
  - Routine FBC, U&Es, thyroid function, autoantibody screen, hepatitis serology, serum ACE, HIV, beta human chorionic gonadotropin (βhCG).
- Respiratory:
  - 6MWT, ABG (room air), overnight oximetry.
  - Pulmonary function tests: typically normal spirometry and lung volumes with reduced diffusing capacity.
- Cardiology:
  - ECG, ECHO, cardiac catheterization.
  - ± Acute pulmonary vaso-reactivity studies using inhaled NO or IV epoprostenol/adenosine:
    - Responder (around 25%): mPAP drop ≥10 mmHg to <40 mmHg.
- Radiology:
  - CXR.
  - HRCT chest: parenchymal disease, mosaic perfusion, features of pulmonary venous hypertension.
  - CTPA: enlarged pulmonary arteries, filling defects, enlarged bronchial circulation.
  - Isotope scanning: more sensitive than CTPA for chronic thromboembolism; not helpful if there is parenchymal lung disease.
  - Selective pulmonary angiography.
  - Cardiac MRI.

Poor prognostic indicators

- Clinical evidence of RV failure, rapid progression of symptoms, syncope, WHO functional class IV, 6MWT <300 m, peak oxygen consumption on exercise testing <12 ml/min/kg, elevated or rising BNP, right atrial pressure >15 mmHg or cardiac index <2.0 L/min/m², extremes of age (<14 or >65 years).

Treatment

- General:
  - Avoid pregnancy (>30% maternal mortality):
    - Progesterone-only contraception or sterilization.
  - Immunizations: pneumococcal/influenza.
  - Supervised exercise rehabilitation, avoiding excess physical activity.
  - Psychosocial support.
- Supportive therapy:
  - Diuretics: if evidence of RV failure/fluid retention.
  - Oxygen: if PaO_2 consistently <8 kPa.
  - Oral anticoagulation.
  - Digoxin.
- Specific drug therapy:
  - Vasoreactive:
    - Calcium channel blockers: high dose nifedipine/diltiazem/amlodipine:
      - Complications: hypotension, peripheral oedema.
  - Non-vasoreactive:
    - Prostaglandin analogues: epoprostenol/iloprost/treprostinil:
      - Complications: flushing, headache, diarrhoea, arthralgia; complications of tunnelled lines.
    - Endothelin receptor antagonists: bosentan, sitaxsentan, ambrisentan:
      - Complications: raised hepatic transaminases.
    - Phosphodiesterase inhibitors: sildenafil, tadalafil:
      - Complications: headache, flushing, epistaxis.
    - Continuous inhaled NO.
- Surgical intervention:
  - Pulmonary endarterectomy: beneficial in chronic thromboembolism.
  - Atrial septostomy: right-to-left shunt; avoid in severe LV failure.
  - Lung transplantation.

Pulmonary vasculitis (*ANCA positive)

Classification

- Small vessel:
  - Wegener's granulomatosis*, Churg–Strauss*, microscopic polyangitis*.
- Medium vessel:
  - Polyarteritis nodosa, Kawasaki disease.
- Large vessel:
  - Giant cell arteritis, Takayasu's arteritis.
- Primary immune complex:
  - Goodpasture's syndrome, Henoch–Schönlein purpura, Behçet's disease, IgA nephropathy.
- Secondary vasculitis:
  - Classic autoimmune disease (systemic lupus erythematosus (SLE), RA, poly/dermatomyositis, scleroderma, antiphospholipid syndrome), cryoglobulinaemia.
- Inflammatory bowel disease.
- Drug induced:
  - A form of hypersensitivity pneumonitis.

+ E.g. nitrofurantoin, sulfonamides, penicillins, phenytoin, propylthiouracil.
- Paraneoplastic.
- Infection:
  + Bacterial superantigens stimulate immune response; ANCA production due to molecular mimicry.

ANCA positive vasculitis:

+ Wegener's granulomatosis:
  - Triad of upper airway disease, lower respiratory tract disease and glomerulonephritis.
  - Alveolar or interstitial infiltrates; nodular or cavitatory disease.
  - Pathologically characterized by a necrotizing small vessel vasculitis, granulomatous inflammation, and parenchymal necrosis.
  - C-ANCA positive in 75–90%.
  - Differential: sarcoidosis, TB, malignancy, Goodpasture's disease, SLE.
+ Churg–Strauss:
  - Triad of asthma, hypereosinophilia, and necrotizing vasculitis.
  - Pulmonary haemorrhage and glomerulonephritis less common than with other ANCA positive vasculitides.
  - P-ANCA positive in 35–75%.
+ Microscopic polyangiitis:
  - Universal glomerulonephritis with pulmonary involvement in 30%.
  - Lung involvement most commonly presents as diffuse alveolar haemorrhage.
  - Often associated with joint, skin, peripheral nerve, and GI involvement.
  - P-ANCA positive in 50–75% and c-ANCA positive in 10–15%.

Pulmonary-renal syndrome:

+ Diffuse alveolar haemorrhage with glomerulonephritis.
+ Differential includes ANCA-associated vasculitis, Goodpasture's syndrome, SLE.

Investigation of pulmonary vasculitis:

+ Biopsy and ANCA are the mainstay of diagnosis.
+ C-ANCA (anti-proteinase 3): highly sensitive (90–95%) and specific (90%) for active Wegener's disease.
+ P-ANCA (anti-myeloperoxidase): suggestive of Churg–Strauss/microscopic polyangiitis but lacks sensitivity and specificity.

Treatment of pulmonary vasculitis:

+ Remission-induction phase then maintenance phase immunosuppression:
  - Oral prednisolone 1 mg/kg/day for 1 month; taper over 6–12 months.
  - ± Cyclophosphamide 2 mg/kg/day (max. 200 mg/day) for 6–12 months.
+ Plasma exchange may be beneficial in Wegener's disease but not Churg–Strauss.
+ PCP and osteoporosis prophylaxis.

EOSINOPHILIC LUNG DISEASE

Eosinophilic lung disease

- Eosinophilic lung disorders are recognized by elevated numbers of eosinophils in the pulmonary parenchyma, defined by the presence of:
  - ◆ Serum eosinophilia with suggestive radiology.
  - ◆ Tissue eosinophilia on lung biopsy.
  - ◆ Eosinophilia on BAL.
- Normal serum eosinophil level <0.4 × 10^9/L; normal BAL eosinophil level <5%.

Parasitic infections

Loeffler's syndrome/simple pulmonary eosinophilia

- Acute response to larvae of helminth (*Strongyloides*, *Ascaris*, *Ankylostoma*) parasites ingested from infected soil, migrating through lungs.
- Features: asymptomatic or brief (up to 14 days) illness with cough, wheeze, dyspnoea, fever, and night sweats.
- Investigation: serum eosinophils normal or mildly elevated; sputum eosinophilia plus larvae on microscopy; stool positive for ova/parasites after 2–3 months; CXR: transient pulmonary infiltrates.
- Treatment: antihelminthic agents (e.g. mebendazole/albendazole for 3 days) if symptomatic.

Tropical pulmonary eosinophilia

- Immune response to infection with filarial worms (*Wuchereria bancrofti*, *Brugia malayi*), transmitted by mosquito vector (India, Asia, Pacific).
- Features: several weeks of cough, wheeze, dyspnoea, fever, weight loss, and lymphadenopathy; waxes and wanes; may develop chronic inflammation and pulmonary fibrosis despite treatment.
- Investigation: marked serum and sputum eosinophilia; raised serum IgE; raised filarial IgG; CXR: patchy infiltrates ± cavitation and occasionally pleural effusion.
- Treatment: antifilarial agents (e.g. diethylcarbamazine for 3 weeks).

Hypersensitivity reactions

Allergic bronchopulmonary aspergillosis (ABPA)

- A complex hypersensitivity reaction, most common in patients with asthma or cystic fibrosis, in response to colonization of bronchi by *Aspergillus*.
- Features: symptoms of poorly controlled asthma, cough, mucous plugs ± haemoptysis, fever, malaise.

- Investigation: serum eosinophilia; raised serum total IgE and *Aspergillus* specific IgE; ± positive *Aspergillus* precipitins (IgG); ± *Aspergillus* on sputum culture; CXR: flitting pulmonary infiltrates ± central bronchiectasis.
- Treatment: prolonged steroids (3–6 months) ± itraconazole.

Drug-induced pulmonary eosinophilia

- Most commonly due to non-steroidal anti-inflammatory drugs (NSAIDs) and antibiotics (nitrofurantoin, sulphonamides, penicillin) but also with antiepileptics, antidepressants, etc.
- Features: onset hours to days after exposure; cough, fever, dyspnoea ± rash; varied course, may progress to respiratory failure.
- Investigation: serum eosinophils often normal; sputum and tissue eosinophilia.
- Treatment: remove precipitant.

Eosinophilic syndromes

Acute eosinophilic pneumonia

- Cause unknown. Male predominance, onset age 20–30 years.
- Features: acute febrile illness (< 7 days' duration), cough, hypoxia, ± respiratory failure requiring ventilation.
- Investigation: serum eosinophils normal (sequestered to lungs); BAL eosinophils >25%; CXR: interstitial/alveolar infiltrates.
- Treatment: high-dose steroids; usually rapid resolution; relapse rare.

Chronic eosinophilic pneumonia

- Cause unknown. Female predominance (2:1), onset in middle age, non-smokers.
- Features: chronic (weeks to months) cough, wheeze, progressive dyspnoea, fever, night sweats, weight loss; often associated with asthma.
- Investigation: serum eosinophils normal or mildly elevated; sputum eosinophilia; CXR: dense peripheral/pleural infiltrates ('inverse pulmonary oedema').
- Treatment: prolonged steroids; relapse common.

Hypereosinophilic syndrome

- Rare. A diagnosis of exclusion—rule out reactive eosinophilia and leukaemia.
- Features: multiorgan involvement; pulmonary disease causes cough, wheeze, pulmonary oedema, pleural effusions, and pulmonary emboli (hypercoagulable).
- Investigation: serum eosinophils > 1.5×10^9/L; often anaemic; eosinophilic infiltrates in muscle, lung, heart, skin, and GI tract on histology.
- Treatment: high-dose steroids and immunosuppressants; prognosis poor.

Miscellaneous

- Churg–Strauss: see Chapter 8: Pulmonary vascular disease.
- Peripheral and/or pulmonary eosinophilic infiltration rarely occurs with primary lung tumours, lung metastases, lymphoma, and acute eosinophilic leukaemia.
- BAL eosinophilia is recognized in idiopathic pulmonary fibrosis, sarcoidosis, hypersensitivity pneumonitis, and connective tissue disorders.

Sleep-disordered breathing

Symptoms

- Daytime somnolence, unrefreshing sleep, morning headaches, impaired concentration, short-term memory loss, personality change, sexual dysfunction, nocturnal choking, snoring, nocturia.
- The Epworth Sleepiness Score (ESS) asks the subject to score their likelihood of falling asleep on a scale of increasing probability from 0 to 3 for 8 different situations:
  - Total score >10, or sleepiness in dangerous situations, even with a normal ESS, warrants sleep evaluation.
  - ESS validated for obstructive sleep apnoea (OSA), and narcolepsy.

Differential diagnoses

- OSA: most common—pharyngeal collapse results from smooth muscle relaxation during sleep, occluding the upper airway:
  - OSA *syndrome*: OSA with sleep fragmentation sufficient to cause symptoms.
- Central sleep apnoea: a cessation or decrease in ventilatory effort during sleep ± wakefulness. Often related to cerebrovascular, cardiac, or neurological disease.
- Mixed sleep apnoea: when OSA is severe and long-standing, central apnoea may develop. May also arise with chronic opiate use.

Risk factors for OSA

- Male sex, age ≥40 yrs, peri-menopause, BMI >30 kg/m^2, collar size ≥16 inches in women or 17 inches in men, micro/retrognathia, abnormal pharyngeal anatomy, nasal congestion (2× risk), diabetes (3× risk), hypothyroidism, acromegaly, sedative medication, excess alcohol, positive family history.

Investigation

- Diagnosis of OSA is based on symptoms and assessment of ventilation during sleep.
- Polysomnography comprises electroencephalography (EEG), electromyography, thoracoabdominal movements, oronasal airflow, pulse oximetry, electrocardiography, sound/video recording:
  - Limited sleep studies are adequate for diagnosis.
  - Overnight oximetry alone may be used as a screening tool.
- Interpretation of polysomnography:
  - Apnoea: an interval ≥10 secs between breaths.
  - Hypopnoea: a period ≥10 secs in which airflow is reduced ≥50% from baseline.
  - Apnoea-hypopnoea index (AHI): the number of episodes of apnoea/hypopnoea per hour. Correlates with the degree of OSA:

- AHI 5–14: mild OSA.
- AHI 15–30: moderate OSA.
- AHI >30: severe OSA.
- Evidence suggests treatment may be beneficial in symptomatic patients with an AHI >15 or a 4% oxygen saturation dip rate at the level of >10/hr.

Reference: Scottish Intercollegiate Guidelines Network 2003.

Management
- Lifestyle modification:
  - ◆ Weight loss if indicated, alcohol restriction, smoking cessation, sleep hygiene, sleep in lateral position or head up 30 degrees.
  - ◆ Advise patients with suspected/confirmed OSA not to drive whilst sleepy:
    - Patients with confirmed OSA must inform the DVLA.
    - Class 2 drivers (large goods vehicle or passenger carrying vehicle, i.e. coaches) require verification of successful treatment by a specialist.
- Mild OSA:
  - ◆ Mandibular advancement device.
  - ◆ Nocturnal CPAP: *only* if symptoms restrict activities of daily living *and* lifestyle modification is inappropriate/unsuccessful.
- Moderate/severe OSA:
  - ◆ Nocturnal CPAP.
  - ◆ Stimulant medication, e.g. modafinil.
  - ◆ Surgery:
    - Very limited supporting evidence; rarely used.
    - Correction of deviated nasal septum, tonsillectomy, adenoidectomy, uvulopalatopharyngo-plasty, tracheostomy, bariatric surgery.
    - Soft palate implants are not recommended by NICE.

Reference: Scottish Intercollegiate Guidelines Network, 2003/ Driver and Vehicle Licensing Agency Guidelines 2011.

Complications of sleep apnoea
- Hypertension, arrhythmia, myocardial infarction, stroke, obesity, diabetes mellitus, pulmonary hypertension.

Obesity hypoventilation (Pickwickian) syndrome
- Can only be diagnosed in the absence of other causes of hypoventilation.
- Characterized by obesity (BMI $\geq$30 kg/m^2), chronic hypercapnia (PaCO$_2$ >6 kPa), and sleep disordered breathing.
- Approximately 90% of patients also have OSA.
- Management: nocturnal CPAP.

Other causes of daytime somnolence
- Idiopathic insomnia, circadian rhythm disorders (shift work/jet lag), neurological disorders (post head injury/encephalitis/parkinsonism), narcolepsy, nocturnal limb movement disorders, stimulant/alcohol dependency sleep disorders, hypothyroidism.

Narcolepsy

- Excessive somnolence with recurrent lapses into sleep almost daily for ≥3 months.
- Associated with:
  - ◆ Cataplexy: sudden loss of bilateral muscle tone provoked by strong emotion.
  - ◆ Sleep paralysis: hypnagogic (at onset of sleep) or hypnopompic (on waking).
  - ◆ Hypnagogic hallucinations: visual, auditory, tactile, or kinetic.
- Treat with stimulants (e.g. modafinil/dexamphetamine) and antidepressants.

Periodic limb movement disorder (PLMD)

- Involuntary limb movement during non-REM (rapid eye movement) sleep.
- Most commonly affects lower limbs:
  - ◆ Partial flexion of the hip, knee, and ankle flexion and great toe extension.
- Diagnosis is by polysomnography:
  - ◆ PLMD: the number of movements per hour of sleep. An index ≥5 is considered abnormal.
- Treat with dopaminergic agents (e.g. ropinirole) to relieve movement disorder and sedatives (e.g. benzodiazepines) to improve sleep quality.
- Distinct from restless leg syndrome (RLS) which is a voluntary response to a sensation of discomfort and typically occurs prior to sleep onset:
  - ◆ 30% of people with PLMD have RLS; 80% of people with RLS have PLMD.
  - ◆ Management of RLS:
    - ▪ Lifestyle modification (avoid caffeine, tobacco, alcohol, and smoking; regular exercise; sleep hygiene).
    - ▪ Replace iron stores if deficient.
    - ▪ Medication as for PLMD plus low-potency opioids and gabapentin.

Mediastinal masses

- Anterior—anterior to the pericardium:
  - The 4Ts: thyroid, thymoma, teratoma (germ cell tumours), terrible lymphoma.
  - Parathyroid tumour.
  - Ascending aortic aneurysm.
  - Morgagni diaphragmatic hernia: antero-medial.
- Middle—bounded by the pericardium, the posterior pericardial reflection, the diaphragm, and the thoracic inlet:
  - Bronchogenic cyst/tumour.
  - Pericardial cyst.
  - Lymphoma.
  - Lymph node hyperplasia.
- Posterior—bounded by the posterior pericardial reflection, the posterior vertebral bodies, the diaphragm, and the first rib:
  - Descending aortic aneurysm.
  - Foregut duplication/gastroenteric cyst.
  - Neurogenic tumour:
    - Sympathetic ganglia (neuroblastoma).
    - Nerve roots (schwannoma/neurofibroma).
  - Bochdalek diaphragmatic hernia: postero-lateral.

Pleural masses

- Radiological features:
  - Smooth, tapered border with obtuse pleural angle.
  - Differ from pulmonary masses which have ill-defined borders, heterogenous opacification, and acute pleural angles.
- Causes:
  - Single mass:
    - Infection: *Actinomycosis, Aspergillosis, Nocardiosis, Blastomycosis, TB.*
    - Malignancy: primary bone tumour, myeloma, lymphoma, metastasis.
    - Haemangioma/haematoma.
    - Lipoma.
  - Multiple masses:
    - Malignancy: metastases (most commonly adenocarcinoma, especially breast).
    - Asbestos-related pleural plaques.

- ◆ Diffuse pleural thickening:
  - ▪ Dose-related response to asbestos exposure with visceral pleural fibrosis.
  - ▪ Mesothelioma.
  - ▪ Malignancy: most commonly adenocarcinoma.
- ◆ Rounded atelectasis:
  - ▪ Also known as shrinking pleuritis/folded lung.
  - ▪ Occurs with chronic pleural scarring, e.g. asbestos-related disease and TB.
  - ▪ Contracting visceral pleural fibrosis incarcerates underlying lung, pulling bronchovascular bundles into the mass; comet tail sign on CT.
  - ▪ Mimics malignancy.

Pleural calcification

- True: asbestos-related pleural plaques, post haemothorax/empyema/TB pleuritis.
- Magnesium mimicking calcification: talc pleurodesis, talcosis.

Pneumothorax

- Risk factors:
  - ◆ Primary: smoking (80–90%), male (6:1 male to female), tall thin habitus, familial (<10%).
  - ◆ Secondary: COPD (60%), asthma, CF, LAM, LCH, ILD, malignancy, pneumonia (fungal, caseating, HIV), TB, Marfan's syndrome, catamenial pneumothorax.
- Diagnosis:
  - ◆ Postero-anterior (PA) chest radiograph (inspiratory).
  - ◆ Lateral radiograph if PA radiograph normal but clinical suspicion high.
  - ◆ CT to differentiate pneumothorax from complex bullous disease.
- Management
  - ◆ Quantify size of pneumothorax on CXR: <2 cm small, ≥2 cm large.
  - ◆ Measure horizontally at level of hilum from lung margin to chest wall.
  - ◆ Breathlessness or haemodynamic instability should prompt intervention, regardless of pneumothorax size.
  - ◆ For management purposes, secondary pneumothoraces are those occurring in patients aged >50 years with a significant smoking history or with underlying lung disease.
  - ◆ Primary:
    - ▪ <2 cm with no breathlessness:
      - ▸ High-flow oxygen.
      - ▸ Discharge with early outpatient review (2–4 weeks).
    - ▪ >2 cm and/or breathlessness:
      - ▸ High-flow oxygen.
      - ▸ Aspirate via 16–18-g cannula; do not exceed 2.5 L total aspirate.
      - ▸ If successful, discharge after 4–6 hrs.
      - ▸ If persistent pneumothorax >2 cm or breathlessness, avoid repeat aspiration and insert intercostal drain.
  - ◆ Secondary:
    - ▪ Admit all patients with secondary pneumothorax for ≥24 hrs.
    - ▪ <1 cm with no breathlessness:
      - ▸ High-flow oxygen (unless risk of CO_2 retention).

- ■ 1–2 cm with no breathlessness:
  - ► High-flow oxygen.
  - ► Aspirate.
  - ► If successful, observe for 24 hrs.
  - ► If persistent pneumothorax >1 cm, insert intercostal drain.
- ■ >2 cm and/or breathlessness:
  - ► High-flow oxygen.
  - ► Insert intercostal drain.
- ■ Remove intercostal drain 24 hrs after re-expansion without clamping.
- ■ Consider high-volume, low-pressure (10–20 cmH$_2$O) suction after 48 hrs if there is a persistent air leak or failure of re-expansion.
- ■ Refer for thoracic surgical opinion after 48 hrs in non-resolving secondary pneumothorax; otherwise refer after 3–5 days.
- ■ Early, aggressive treatment recommended in CF and HIV.
- ■ Encourage smoking cessation in all patients.
- ■ For guidance regarding air travel/diving see Chapter 12: Environmental lung disease.

Reference: British Thoracic Society Guidelines 2010.

- • Indications for surgery:
  - ◆ 1st contralateral pneumothorax or 2nd ipsilateral pneumothorax.
  - ◆ Bilateral spontaneous pneumothorax.
  - ◆ Persistent air leak.
  - ◆ Spontaneous haemothorax.
  - ◆ Professions at risk, e.g. pilots/divers.
  - ◆ Medical pleurodesis only indicated in patients unwilling or unfit for surgery.

Recurrence rate without definitive management (after 1st episode):

- ◆ Most common within first 6 months to 2 years.
- ◆ Primary pneumothorax: range 16–52%, average 30%.
- ◆ Secondary pneumothorax: range 39–47%, up to 90% in CF.

Recurrence rate with definitive management:

- ◆ Open thoracotomy and pleurectomy: <0.5%.
- ◆ VATS: 5–10%. Chemical pleurodesis: talc 9% (risk of empyema/ARDS), tetracycline 16%.

Tension pneumothorax:

- ◆ Risk factors: non-invasive/invasive ventilation, trauma, CPR, chest drain occlusion/displacement, acute asthma, and COPD.
- ◆ Management: high-flow oxygen, emergency needle decompression, and intercostal drain.

Unilateral pleural effusion

- • Diagnosis:
  - ◆ Aspirate under US guidance.
  - ◆ Do not aspirate if effusion bilateral and clinical findings suggest transudate.
  - ◆ Send aspirate for protein, LDH, Gram stain, acid-alcohol fast bacilli (AAFB), culture and cytology.

- ◆ ± pH: normally 7.6; low in empyema, RA, and oesophageal rupture (<6).
- ◆ ± Glucose: low in empyema and RA (<1.6 mmol/L).
- ◆ ± Amylase with iso-enzymes: raised in pancreatitis and oesophageal rupture.
- ◆ ± Triglycerides and chylomicrons: chylothorax (trauma, malignancy, LAM).
- ◆ ± Cholesterol crystals: pseudochylothorax (TB, RA).
- ◆ ± Creatinine: raised in urinothorax.
- ◆ ± Haematocrit: >50% blood haematocrit in haemothorax.
- ◆ ± Complement: C4 low in RA.
- ◆ Pleural fluid tumour markers are poorly sensitive and not currently recommended.
- If aspiration non-diagnostic:
  - ◆ Contrast-enhanced CT chest.
  - ◆ Pleural biopsy: if suspicion of pleural malignancy or TB:
    - ■ Image-guided cutting needle recommended over Abram's needle.
  - ◆ Thoracoscopy/VATS.
  - ◆ Bronchoscopy: if haemoptysis or suspicion of bronchial obstruction.
- Transudate—protein <25 g/L:
  - ◆ Left ventricular failure, cirrhotic liver disease (hepatic hydrothorax), hypo-albuminaemia, peritoneal dialysis, hypothyroidism, Meig's syndrome.
- Exudate—protein >35 g/L:
  - ◆ Malignancy, mesothelioma, infection, pulmonary infarction, RA, SLE, oesophageal rupture, pancreatitis, drug-induced.
- Light's criteria for exudative effusion—use if protein 25–35 g/L:
  - ◆ Ratio of pleural fluid to serum protein >0.5.
  - ◆ Ratio of pleural fluid to serum LDH >0.6.
  - ◆ Pleural fluid LDH >2/3 of the upper limit of normal serum value.
- Neutrophilic:
  - ◆ Any acute effusion, commonly parapneumonic, pulmonary infarction.
- Lymphocytic:
  - ◆ Chronic effusions, TB, malignancy, lymphoma, RA, sarcoidosis.
- Eosinophilic:
  - ◆ Haemothorax, pneumothorax, malignancy, infection (fungal and parasitic), drug-induced, asbestos-induced, Churg–Strauss syndrome, post-coronary artery bypass graft (CABG).
- Indications for drainage:
  - ◆ Purulent fluid on aspiration.
  - ◆ Positive Gram stain or culture.
  - ◆ Pleural fluid pH <7.2.
  - ◆ Loculated effusion.
  - ◆ Large effusion with associated dyspnoea.

Pleural infection

- Risk factors:
  - ◆ Immunosuppression including corticosteroids, diabetes mellitus, gastro-oesophageal reflux, alcohol/IV drug abuse.
- Natural history:
  - ◆ Parapneumonic effusion (exudate) due to increased capillary permeability.

- ◆ Fibropurulent stage with bacterial invasion.
- ◆ Organizing stage with fibroblast proliferation and formation of pleural rind.
- Microbiology (in order of descending frequency):
  - ◆ Community acquired:
    - *Streptococcus: S. milleri, S. pneumoniae, S. intermedius.*
    - *Staphylococcus aureus.*
    - Gram negative anaerobes: *Enterobacter, Escherichia coli.*
    - Anaerobes: *Fusobacterium, Bacteroides, Peptostreptococcus*, mixed.
  - ◆ Hospital acquired:
    - Staphylococci: MRSA, *S. aureus.*
    - Gram negative anaerobes: *E. coli, Pseudomonas, Klebsiella.*
    - Anaerobes.
- Blood cultures indicated in all cases of suspected pleural infection—positive in 14%.
- Management
  - ◆ Thromboprophylaxis.
  - ◆ Nutritional supplementation to avoid hypoalbuminaemia.
  - ◆ Intercostal drainage.
  - ◆ Antibiotics universally indicated in pleural infection:
    - Ideally, guided by culture results and local policy.
    - Empirical therapy for community-acquired infection:
      - ▸ Penicillin (±β lactamase inhibitor) plus metronidazole.
      - ▸ Penicillin allergic: clindamycin ± ciprofloxacin/cephalosporin.
      - ▸ Avoid aminoglycosides which have poor pleural penetration.
      - ▸ Macrolides not indicated unless suspicion of atypical infection.
    - Empirical therapy for hospital-acquired infection should cover MRSA.
    - Duration of antibiotics often ≥3 weeks.
  - ◆ Intrapleural antibiotics and fibrinolytics not recommended.
  - ◆ Refer for thoracic surgical opinion if there is persistent sepsis with a pleural collection despite chest drainage and antibiotics.
  - ◆ Surgical options:
    - VATS (first line).
    - Rib resection and placement of large-bore drain.
    - Thoracotomy and decortications.
- Note: small-bore drains (10–14 F) recommended as first line for pneumothorax, free flowing effusions, and pleural infection. Use 28–30 F for haemothorax.

Reference: British Thoracic Society Guidelines 2010.

OCCUPATIONAL AND ENVIRONMENTAL LUNG DISEASE

Causes of occupational lung disease

- Coal dust exposure (coal mining):
  - COPD: increased frequency in coal miners.
  - Pneumoconiosis (simple):
    - Nodules <1 cm, upper and middle zones on CXR.
    - Relatively benign disease.
  - Progressive massive fibrosis (PMF or complicated pneumoconiosis):
    - Nodules >1 cm, mostly upper zones.
    - Associated emphysema, cavities, necrosis, calcification.
  - Caplan's syndrome:
    - Bilateral peripheral nodules ± cavities with rheumatoid factor seropositivity.
    - Benign prognosis; mostly asymptomatic.
- Beryllium exposure (manufacture of electrical parts, mining):
  - Berylliosis:
    - Acute inhalation of fumes: pulmonary oedema and alveolitis.
    - Skin exposure or inhalation: hypersensitivity reaction with non-caseating granulomas and progressive fibrosis (sarcoid-like).
- Silica exposure (foundry work, sandblasting, stone cutting, mining):
  - Silicosis: a spectrum of disease:
    - Acute high-level exposure: progressive bi-basal fibrosis.
    - Lower level exposure: upper and mid zone nodules ± PMF, egg-shell calcification of hilar lymph nodes, ± pleural thickening.
    - Increased risk of active MTB and NTM infections.
  - Silicosis- like picture also occurs with iron oxide from welding (siderosis), aluminium, tin, and barium.
- Asbestos exposure (mining, pipe lagging, insulation, restoration work):
  - Asbestos fibre types:
    - Serpentine: chrysotile (white)—the most commonly used and least pathogenic fibre type.
    - Amphibole: crocidolite (blue), amosite (brown), anthophyllite, etc.
  - Mining and use now highly restricted, peak industrial exposure was in the 1970s.
  - Asbestosis:
    - Fibrosis associated with asbestos exposure; dose related.
    - Latent period 20–30 years.
    - Dry cough, progressive dyspnoea, and respiratory failure.
    - An independent risk factor for lung cancer.
    - Management: nil specific, smoking cessation, cancer surveillance.

- Asbestos plaques:
  - A marker of exposure to asbestos; latent period 20–40 years.
  - Circumscribed, discrete areas of hyaline or calcified fibrosis.
  - May develop exudative pleural effusions which wax and wane; usually unilateral; exclude TB and malignancy.
  - Management: smoking cessation.
- Diffuse pleural thickening:
  - Dose related.
  - Exertional dyspnoea and chest pain.
  - Smooth, non-interrupted, plural thickening, often extending into costophrenic angles with adhesions and loss of the pleural space.
- Rounded atelectasis:
  - See Chapter 11: Disorders of the mediastinum and pleura.
- Asbestos-related lung cancer:
  - Asbestos exposure increases lung cancer risk by up to 5 times.
  - Smoking and asbestos combined increase risk by 80–90 times.
- Mesothelioma:
  - No relation to asbestos dose or smoking.
  - Latent period 30–40 years.
  - Aggressive pleural malignancy with irregular thickening and nodularity on CT.
  - Local extension to mediastinum and peritoneal pleura.
  - Chest pain, dyspnoea, large unilateral pleural effusions.
  - Median survival 8–14 months.
  - Palliative care options include early pleurodesis, debulking surgery, radiotherapy for aspiration sites and pain relief, chemotherapy (limited results).

Occupational asthma

- Under-reported; accounts for up to 1 in 10 cases of adult-onset asthma.
- Most common precipitants:
  - Flour, grain dust, wood dust, isocyanates, colophony and fluxes, latex, aldehydes, animals.
- Increased risk in atopic individuals.
- Occupation asthma often preceded by occupational rhinitis.
- Preventative measures:
  - Workplace risk assessment and exposure control for possible asthmagens.
  - Health surveillance for early disease detection/removal from exposure.
  - Serial peak flow measurements are highly sensitive and specific; measure every 2 hrs during waking hours for 4 continuous weeks.
- Management:
  - Complete removal from exposure, the earlier the better, ideally within 1 year of symptom onset.
  - If symptoms persist, treatment the same as non-occupational asthma.

Reference: British Thoracic Society Guidelines 2008.

Compensation for occupational lung disease

- Common law claim:
  - ◆ Action against firm where exposure occurred.
  - ◆ Must occur within 3 years of diagnosis.
- Pneumoconiosis etc. Workers' Compensation Act (1979):
  - ◆ For individuals unable to claim damages from the employer responsible because they have ceased trading; one-off, lump-sum payout.
- Industrial Injuries Disablement Benefit:
  - ◆ For 'prescribed diseases' recognized by Department of Work & Pensions.
  - ◆ COPD, occupational rhinitis, occupational asthma, pneumoconiosis, byssinosis, diffuse pleural thickening, mesothelioma, lung cancer (when accompanied by asbestosis or diffuse pleural thickening).
- War pension: if exposure occurred during military service.

Hypersensitivity pneumonitis

- See Chapter 7: Interstitial lung disease.

Environmental lung disease

Flight

- Most large aircraft compress cabin to ≈2400 m; partial pressure of oxygen reduced by 25% (equivalent to FiO_2 15%) and gas volumes increased by 30%.
- In those with normal lungs, oxygen saturations are 85–91% (PaO_2 7–8.5 kPa).
- In those with underlying lung disease hypoxia is exacerbated.

Reference: British Thoracic Society Guidelines 2011.

- Historical recommendations for in-flight oxygen in patients with lung disease
  - ◆ Sats* >95%: no oxygen required.
  - ◆ Sats* 92–95%: consider hypoxic challenge testing (15% FiO_2 for 15 min)—oxygen required if PaO_2 <6.6 kPa.
  - ◆ Sats* <92%: oxygen required.
  - ◆ (*At rest, on air, at sea level)

Reference: British Thoracic Society Guidelines 2004.

- Updated BTS guidance recognizes neither resting saturations nor FEV_1 reliably predict hypoxaemia or in-flight complications, and advises a pragmatic approach.
- If normally on oxygen, increase flow rate (max 4 L/min).
- Pneumothorax:
  - ◆ Spontaneous: fit to fly 7 days after complete resolution (radiological).
  - ◆ Traumatic: fit to fly 2 weeks after complete resolution.
  - ◆ If surgical pleurodesis, can travel once recovered from surgery.
- PTB:
  - ◆ Fit to fly 2 weeks after starting treatment.
  - ◆ HIV positive need 3 negative smears or negative culture.

Diving

- For every 10-m descent, ambient pressure increases by 100 kPa (1 bar).
- Gas volume is inversely proportional to pressure resulting in compression on descent and expansion on ascent.
- Barotrauma: 'pressure trauma':
  - Descent: alveolar exudation and haemorrhage.
  - Ascent: alveolar rupture, pneumothorax, pneumomediastinum, arterial gas embolism.
- Decompression illness:
  - Intravascular or extravascular bubbles, especially nitrogen, form as environmental pressure reduces with ascent (decompression).
  - Manifestations include itching, paraesthesiae, joint pains, neurological symptoms, cardiovascular collapse, and death.
  - Risk increased in asthma, COPD (gas trapping), and patent foramen ovale.
  - Management: 100% oxygen ± recompression.
- Fitness to dive:
  - Spirometry should be measured in all patients with CXR ± CT chest for those with a history of lung disease.
- Contraindications to diving:
  - Untreated pneumothorax, CF, active sarcoidosis, active TB, bullous lung disease, exercise-induced or poorly controlled asthma.
- Pneumothorax:
  - Spontaneous: cannot dive unless bilateral surgical pleurectomy, normal PFTs and CT chest post-surgery.
  - Traumatic pneumothorax: may dive if healed with normal PFTs (including flow volume loop) and CT chest.
- Asthma:
  - Subjects with asthma may be permitted to dive if they are asymptomatic with normal spirometry (FEV_1 >80% predicted; FEV_1/FVC >70%) and a negative exercise test (<15% fall in FEV_1).
  - Diving should be avoided in patients requiring relief medication in the preceding 48 hrs, with a fall in PEFR ≥10% from best and with diurnal PEFR variability ≥20%.

Reference: British Thoracic Society Guidelines 2003.

Chapter 13

LUNG TRANSPLANTATION

Indications

- The most common diagnoses resulting in lung transplant are COPD, IPF, CF, idiopathic pulmonary hypertension, and A1AT deficiency.
- In general, patients should be referred for transplant assessment if their predicted 2–3-yr survival is <50% and/or they are New York Heart Association (NYHA) functional class III or IV.
- Disease-specific referral criteria are detailed as follows:

Table 13.1 Disease-specific transplantation criteria

Disease	Indications for transplant referral	Indications for transplantation
Bronchiectasis/ cystic fibrosis	FEV_1 <30% predicted or rapidly declining Increasing frequency or severity of exacerbations Refractory and/or recurrent pneumothorax Recurrent haemoptysis despite embolization	Oxygen-dependent respiratory failure Hypercapnia Pulmonary hypertension
COPD	BODE index >5	BODE index 7–10 and any of: Admission with acute hypercapnia Pulmonary hypertension and/or cor pulmonale despite LTOT FEV_1 <20% predicted and either TLCO <20% predicted or homogenous emphysema
Pulmonary fibrosis	Histological or radiographic evidence of usual interstitial pneumonia (UIP) Histological evidence of fibrotic NSIP	Histological or radiographic evidence of UIP and any of: TLCO <39% predicted Fall in FVC ≥10% over 6 months Desaturation to <88% during 6MWT Honeycombing on HRCT (fibrosis score of >2) Histological evidence of NSIP and any of: TLCO <35% predicted Fall in FVC ≥10% or fall in TLCO ≥15% over 6 months
Pulmonary arterial hypertension	NYHA functional class III or IV Rapidly progressive disease	Persistent NYHA class III or IV despite maximal medical therapy Failure of infused medical therapy 6MWT <350 m or falling Cardiac index <2 L/min/m2 Right atrial pressure >15 mmHg

Reference: International Society for Heart and Lung Transplantation Guidelines 2006.

Contraindications

- Absolute:
  - ◆ Significant chest wall/spinal deformity.
  - ◆ Untreatable advanced extrapulmonary organ dysfunction.
  - ◆ Non-curable extrapulmonary infection, e.g. chronic active hepatitis B, hepatitis C, HIV.
  - ◆ Malignancy in the last 2 years, excepting squamous/basal cell skin tumours.
  - ◆ Documented non-compliance with medical therapy and/or follow-up.
  - ◆ Untreatable psychiatric illness precluding compliance.
  - ◆ Absence of an adequate social support system.
  - ◆ Substance addiction in the last 6 months (tobacco/alcohol/narcotics).
- Relative:
  - ◆ Age >65 years:
    - Age >50 years for heart–lung; 60 years for double lung; 65 years for single lung.
  - ◆ Unstable or critical condition including mechanical ventilation.
  - ◆ Severely limited functional status with poor rehabilitation potential.
  - ◆ Colonization with highly resistant/virulent bacteria, fungi, or mycobacteria, e.g. *Burkholderia cepacia*, *Aspergillus*.
  - ◆ Severe obesity defined as a BMI ≥30 kg/m^2.
  - ◆ Severe or symptomatic osteoporosis.

Transplant work-up

- FBC, U&Es, liver function, clotting, ABO and HLA phenotyping, creatinine clearance.
- Sputum microscopy, culture, and sensitivity (MC&S), viral serology (HIV, hepatitis B/C, toxoplasmosis, CMV, Epstein–Barr virus (EBV)), tuberculin skin test.
- CXR PA and lateral, CT chest with contrast, ventilation/perfusion (V/Q) scan, DEXA scan.
- ECG, ECHO, myocardial perfusion scintigraphy, left and right heart catheterization.
- Cervical smear, mammography, prostate-specific antigen (PSA), faecal occult blood, colonoscopy.
- Full pulmonary function tests, ABG, 6MWT.

Surgical procedures

- Lobar from live donors:
  - ◆ For patients too ill to await cadaveric transplantation.
  - ◆ Single lobe harvested from each of 2 donors; recipient undergoes bilateral pneumonectomy and implantation.
- Single lung:
  - ◆ Pulmonary fibrosis, older patients with COPD.
  - ◆ Accounts for the majority (50%) of lung transplants performed.
- Double lung:
  - ◆ CF, bronchiectasis, pulmonary hypertension, young patients with COPD.
  - ◆ Most commonly performed sequentially versus en bloc.
- Heart–lung:
  - ◆ Eisenmenger's syndrome, pulmonary hypertension with cor pulmonale, end-stage lung disease with concurrent severe cardiac disease.

◆ In a domino procedure patients without cardiac disease receive a heart–lung transplant because it is technically easier and their heart is donated onwards.

Postoperative care

- Ventilation to avoid hyperoxaemia and barotrauma, bronchial hygiene with suctioning/ bronchoscopy, management of cardiac dysrhythmia, fluid balance to maintain low capillary wedge pressures.
- Immunosuppression:
  ◆ Maintenance triple therapy is standard: combination of tacrolimus, mycophenolate mofetil, and corticosteroids.
  ◆ Tacrolimus: calcineurin inhibitor; side effects of renal dysfunction, hypertension, neurotoxicity, glucose intolerance.
  ◆ Mycophenolate: selective inhibition of B- and T-cell proliferation; side effects of diarrhoea, nausea, vomiting, opportunistic infection; toxic in pregnancy.
  ◆ First-line treatment of rejection is a high-dose IV steroid pulse.
  ◆ For ongoing rejection add rapamycin or antithrombocyte globulin.
- Antimicrobial prophylaxis:
  ◆ Pre-transplant vaccination: *Streptococcus pneumoniae*, tetanus, diphtheria, hepatitis A/B and varicella.
  ◆ Bacterial: broad spectrum ± antipseudomonal cover.
  ◆ Fungal: septrin to cover *Pneumocystis jiroveci*, voriconazole to cover *Aspergillus* ± inhaled amphotericin B.
  ◆ Viral: acyclovir to cover herpes simplex, ganciclovir to cover CMV.

Complications

- Re-perfusion injury:
  ◆ Non-cardiogenic pulmonary oedema.
- Early graft dysfunction:
  ◆ Diffuse alveolar damage due to severe donor lung ischemia, donor lung injury, or vascular anastomotic stenosis.
- Rejection:
  ◆ Hyperacute: occurs within minutes; IgG mediated diffuse alveolar damage.
  ◆ Acute: occurs up to 3 months post transplant; cell-mediated response to graft, lymphocytic infiltration manifests as dyspnoea, fever, leucocytosis, and FEV_1 decrease >10% below baseline. Responds rapidly to corticosteroids and increased immunosuppression.
  ◆ Chronic/bronchiolitis obliterans syndrome: affects 80% within 10 years; lymphocytic infiltration and fibroproliferation lead to airway obstruction non-responsive to corticosteroids/ bronchodilators.
- Infection:
  ◆ Increased risk from immunosuppression, reduced mucociliary clearance, reduced cough reflex due to denervation and loss of lymphatic drainage.
  ◆ Bacterial pneumonias most common, especially Gram negative.
  ◆ CMV is a common cause of viral pneumonia post-transplant.

- Malignancy:
  - Post-transplant lymphoproliferative disorders range from benign polyclonal hyperplasia to high-grade lymphoma:
    - Most commonly B cell; prognosis worse if T cell.
  - EBV may be the causative agent.
  - Treatment is with antiviral agents and reduced immunosuppression.

Outcomes of lung transplantation

- Vary with pre-transplant diagnosis; mean 1-yr survival 78% and 5-yr survival 51%.

INVASIVE AND NON-INVASIVE VENTILATION

Non-invasive ventilation (NIV)

- Pressure-controlled ventilation:
  - Continuous positive airway pressure (CPAP).
  - Bilevel positive airway pressure (BIPAP); also known as NIV.
- Mechanism of action:
  - CPAP: IPAP = EPAP:
    - Positive-end expiratory pressure (PEEP).
  - BIPAP: IPAP > EPAP:
    - PEEP plus pressure support.
- Indications
  - CPAP:
    - Acute hypoxaemic respiratory failure (e.g. severe pneumonia, immunocompromise) or cardiogenic pulmonary oedema refractory to medical therapy.
  - BIPAP:
    - Acute hypercapnic respiratory failure with pH <7.35, pCO_2 >6, or evidence of respiratory distress with raised respiratory rate, e.g. COPD exacerbation, chest wall deformity, neuromuscular weakness, decompensated obesity hypoventilation syndrome.
    - pH <7.26 may be suitable but higher rates of treatment failure.
    - Failure of optimal medical therapy after a maximum 1 hr.
- Contraindications:
  - Impaired consciousness/confusion/cardiorespiratory arrest.
  - Severe hypoxaemia.
  - Haemodynamic instability or life-threatening arrhythmia.
  - Excessive secretions/vomiting.
  - High risk of aspiration/bowel obstruction/upper GI surgery.
  - Facial burns/trauma/surgery/deformity.
  - Untreated pneumothorax.
- Benefits:
  - Reduces intubation rates and mortality in patients with COPD.
- Complications:
  - Facial and nasal pressure injury and sores.
  - Gastric distension and aspiration of gastric contents.
  - Dry mucous membranes and thick secretions.
- BIPAP set-up:
  - Start with full face mask.
  - Initial pressures should be low: IPAP 10, EPAP 5 (cmH2O).
  - Increase IPAP in 2.5–5-cmH2O increments.

- ◆ Usual maximum pressures: IPAP 20, EPAP 4–5 (cmH2O).
- ◆ Entrain oxygen into circuit to maintain saturations (usual target 88–92%).
- ◆ ABGs at 1, 4, and 12 hrs plus 1 hr after changing settings.
- ◆ Continuous pulse oximetry and ECG monitoring for first 12 hrs.
- ◆ Review requirement for escalation to intubation within 4 hrs.
- BIPAP weaning:
  - ◆ Continue BIPAP until resolution of acute pathology, pH ≥7.35 and normal respiratory rate; typically wean over 4 days (initially during daytime).
- Long-term use of BIPAP:
  - ◆ May be useful in chronic hypercapnia and mild hypoxemia.
  - ◆ Neuromuscular/chest wall disease:
    - Effective in muscular dystrophy/kyphoscoliosis/post-polio.
    - Use in motor neuron disease controversial; avoid if bulbar pathology.
  - ◆ Obesity hypoventilation syndrome/decompensated obstructive sleep apnoea.
  - ◆ Cystic fibrosis: used as a bridge to lung transplantation.
  - ◆ Idiopathic pulmonary fibrosis: poor response.

Reference: Royal College of Physicians/ British Thoracic Society Guidelines 2008

Invasive ventilation

- Modes of ventilation:
  - ◆ Volume controlled: set desired tidal volume; inspiratory pressure varies according to pulmonary resistance and compliance.
  - ◆ Pressure controlled: set desired inspiratory pressure; tidal volume varies.
- Trigger variables:
  - ◆ Continuous mandatory ventilation: ventilator triggers all breaths.
  - ◆ Assist control ventilation: patient triggers all breaths.
  - ◆ Intermittent mandatory ventilation: ventilator provides minimum number of breaths but allows patient to trigger a breath at any time.
- PEEP:
  - ◆ Normal airway pressure at the end of expiration is zero; application of pressure at this stage of the ventilatory cycle is known as PEEP.
  - ◆ 'Auto PEEP' is the pressure within the airway on closure of the glottis:
    - In healthy lungs this equates to a PEEP setting of 5 cmH_2O.
    - Gas trapping causes an increase in auto-PEEP.
  - ◆ Therapeutic PEEP levels range from 10–35 cmH_2O.
  - ◆ PEEP prevents airway and alveolar collapse, reducing atelectasis and V/Q mismatch and improving oxygenation.
- Pressure support:
  - ◆ An adjunct to ventilation; usual range 5–30 cmH_2O.
  - ◆ Positive pressure breath delivered at set pressure to support inspiratory effort, increasing tidal volumes and reducing hypercapnia.
  - ◆ Reduces muscular work of breathing; role in weaning.
- Indications for invasive ventilation:
  - ◆ Respiratory failure/exhaustion.
  - ◆ Airway protection: tracheal injury, oedema, head injury, facial fractures.
  - ◆ Airway hygiene: excessive secretions.

- Complications of invasive ventilation:
  - Complications of intubation:
    - Tooth avulsion, upper airway/vocal cord trauma, tracheal laceration/perforation, tube misplacement, hypoxemia.
  - Ventilator-induced lung injury:
    - Volutrauma/barotrauma:
      - Local over-distension of alveoli (preferential ventilation of normal lung) and shear forces cause alveolar epithelial injury, alveolar rupture, pneumothorax (± tension), pneumomediastinum, and acute lung injury/ARDS.
      - Increased risk with large tidal volumes and elevated peak inspiratory and plateau pressures.
      - Effects greater if underlying lung disease or existing ARDS.
    - Prevention/treatment strategies:
      - 'Protective ventilation': low tidal volumes with high PEEP ± permissive hypercapnia (accept pCO_2 >6 with pH >7.15).
      - High-frequency oscillatory ventilation: RR >60 bpm with very small tidal volumes.
  - Oxygen toxicity:
    - Manifestations include tracheobronchitis, atelectasis, hypercarbia, and diffuse alveolar damage/ARDS.
  - Ventilator-associated pneumonia—see Chapter 4: Pulmonary infection.
- Weaning from invasive ventilation:
  - Requires adequate ventilation, oxygenation, and airway.
  - Consider tracheostomy if ventilated for ≥7 days; reduces airway resistance, eases communication, facilitates hygiene and patient comfort.
- Invasive ventilation in asthma/COPD:
  - High PEEP required to overcome auto-PEEP.
  - Prolonged expiratory phase to minimize gas trapping/hyperinflation.
- Other options for oxygenation/CO_2 removal:
  - Extracorporeal membrane oxygenation (ECMO): partial cardiopulmonary bypass; gas exchange occurs by diffusion via an external membrane.

Spirometry and flow volume loops

- Spirometry measures volume against time:
  - FEV$_1$: forced expiratory volume in 1 sec.
  - FVC: forced vital capacity.
  - Ratio of FEV$_1$:FVC (normal ratio >70%).
- Flow volume loops display flow (L/sec) against volume (L):
  - Flow is greatest when the lung volume is greatest, hence the rapid rise to peak expiratory flow rate (PEFR).
  - As volume falls, elastic recoil forces are reduced and airways narrow; flow reduces until the residual volume (RV) is reached.
  - FEF$_{25-75}$%: forced expiratory flow averaged for the middle half of the FVC manoeuvre; a more sensitive but less reproducible measure of medium/small airway narrowing than FEV$_1$.

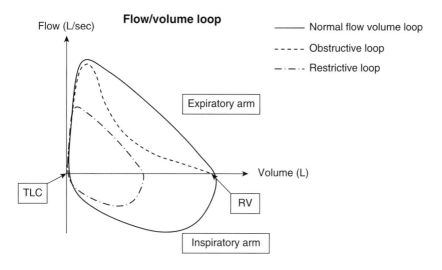

Obstructive spirometry

- Obstructive lung disease: asthma, COPD, A1AT deficiency, bronchiectasis, CF.
- FEV$_1$:FVC ratio <70% with FEV$_1$ <80% predicted:
  - FEV$_1$ falls disproportionately greater than FVC.

- Flow volume loop: concave flattening of expiratory arm ('scalloping'):
  - Flow diminishes during expiration due to airway collapse, reducing lung volumes and increasing resistance.
  - Prolonged time to full expiration but normal inspiratory curve.

Restrictive spirometry

- Restrictive lung disease: interstitial lung disease, pleural disease, neuromuscular disease, diaphragm dysfunction, kyphoscoliosis, obesity, pregnancy.
- FEV_1:FVC ratio >80%:
  - Reduction of FEV_1 *and* FVC.
- Flow volume loop: small but with relatively normal inspiratory/expiratory curves.

Mixed obstructive/restrictive spirometry

- FEV_1:FVC ratio <70% *and* reduction in FVC.
- The result of concurrent lung pathology or airway closure with gas trapping; differentiate according to TLC.

Upper airways obstruction

Fixed upper airways obstruction

- Upper airway pathology that does not vary with inspiration or expiration:
  - Maximal flow rates limited.
- Flow volume loop: characteristic flattening in both inspiration and expiration.
- Causes: tracheal/bronchial stenosis, goitre, upper airway tumours.

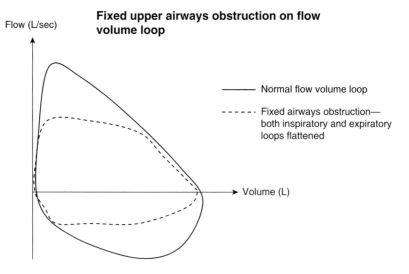

Fixed upper airways obstruction on flow volume loop

Flow (L/sec)

—— Normal flow volume loop

----- Fixed airways obstruction— both inspiratory and expiratory loops flattened

Volume (L)

Variable upper airways obstruction

- Different patterns depend on the level of the narrowing.
- Variable *intrathoracic* obstruction:
  - Inspiration:
    - Decreased intrathoracic pressure splints open the airway lumen at the site of intrathoracic obstruction, maintaining flow.

- Normal inspiratory flow curve.
- Expiration:
  - Increased intrathoracic pressure narrows the airway lumen at the site of intrathoracic obstruction, limiting flow.
  - Flattened expiratory flow curve.
- Causes: tracheomalacia, polychondritis, low tracheal/bronchial tumours.

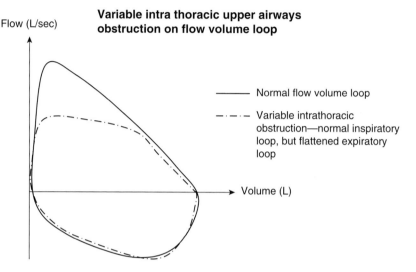

Variable intra thoracic upper airways obstruction on flow volume loop

Flow (L/sec)

——— Normal flow volume loop

—·—·— Variable intrathoracic obstruction—normal inspiratory loop, but flattened expiratory loop

Volume (L)

- Variable *extrathoracic* obstruction:
  - Inspiration:
    - Acceleration of air into the lungs reduces intraluminal pressures causing collapse at the site of extrathoracic obstruction.
    - Flattened inspiratory flow curve.

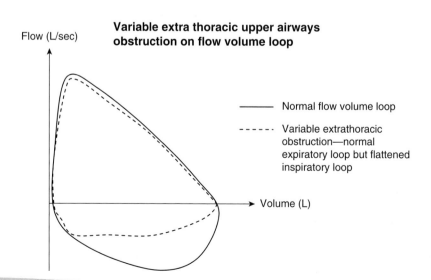

Variable extra thoracic upper airways obstruction on flow volume loop

Flow (L/sec)

——— Normal flow volume loop

----- Variable extrathoracic obstruction—normal expiratory loop but flattened inspiratory loop

Volume (L)

  ◆ Expiration:
    ▪ Expiration forces air via a narrowed (± expandable) extrathoracic airway.
    ▪ Normal expiratory flow curve.
  ◆ Causes: vocal cord paralysis (unilateral/bilateral), airway burns, laryngeal oedema, glottic strictures.

Lung volume measurements

- Volumes: tidal volume (TV), inspiratory reserve volume (IRV), expiratory reserve volume (ERV), residual volume (RV).
- Capacities (comprise ≥2 of the basic lung volumes): total lung capacity (TLC = RV + IRV + ERV + TV), vital capacity (VC = TLC − RV), functional residual capacity (FRC = RV + ERV).

Helium dilution

- Used to measure FRC.
- Patient inhales gas mixture with helium and holds breath for 10 secs.
- Helium distributes throughout airways excluding trapped lung gas.
- Measures only communicating airspaces, not bullae or cavities.
- Distal airway obstruction may therefore result in underestimation of FRC.

Whole-body plethysmography (WBP)

- Patient sits in airtight chamber and makes inspiratory and expiratory effort against a closed valve.
- Measures non-communicating volume as well as communicating volume.
- Difference between WBP and helium dilution indicates volume of bullous disease.

Lung volumes in obstructive lung disease

- Key feature is an increase in RV.
- Air trapping: low VC, normal TLC, high RV and RV:TLC.
- Hyperinflation: normal VC, high TLC, high RV and RV:TLC.

Lung volumes in restrictive lung disease

- Key feature is a decrease in TLC.
- Parenchymal lung disease: reductions in all lung volumes; RV:TLC may remain normal.
- Raised BMI: reductions in all lung volumes, especially FRC and ERV; normal RV:TLC.
- Neuromuscular weakness: low VC, low TLC, high RV and RV:TLC in severe expiratory muscle weakness (may cause confusion with obstructive disorders).

Gas transfer measurements

- TLCO: carbon monoxide transfer factor (mmol/min/kPa).
- KCO: transfer factor corrected for alveolar volume (TLCO/VA).
- VA: alveolar volume.

Carbon monoxide (CO) transfer method

- Patient inhales gas mixture (CO, helium, oxygen, and nitrogen), holds breath for 10 secs and exhales into a sample bag.
- Helium dilution is used to estimate alveolar/total lung volumes.

- CO uptake is measured as a concentration fall in CO and is used to calculate diffusing capacity (TLCO); uptake is limited by both perfusion and diffusion.

Increased TLCO

- Pulmonary haemorrhage, left-to-right shunt, ± acute asthma.

Reduced TLCO

- Anaemia reduces TLCO therefore correct for haematocrit.
- Emphysema, interstitial lung disease, and pulmonary vascular disease:
  - Low TLCO, low KCO.
- Non-pulmonary processes that reduce TLC (e.g. chest wall deformity, neuromuscular weakness, obesity, diffuse pleural thickening, lung resection, small lungs):
  - Low TLCO, normal KCO.

Airway hyper-responsiveness

Reversibility

- Positive if increase in FEV_1 or FVC > 12% or 200 ml to inhaled bronchodilator.

Bronchial provocation tests

- For patients with suspected airway hyper-responsiveness but normal spirometry.
- Direct: agents such as histamine and methacholine act directly on smooth muscle to cause contraction and airway narrowing:
  - Methacholine challenge testing:
    - Methacholine inhaled at increasing concentrations with repeated spirometry.
    - Positive result with fall in FEV_1 >20% (PC_{20}: provocative concentration in mg/mL).
    - Lower PC_{20} indicates lower concentration of methacholine needed to induce bronchospasm so more sensitive airway.
- Indirect: hyperosmolar stimuli or hyperpnoea trigger inflammatory mediator release to indirectly cause smooth muscle contraction.

Exercise testing

Incremental shuttle walk test (ISWT)

- Patient walks 10-m course with increasing speed to keep up with a tape of preset 'bleeps' at decreasing time intervals; no encouragement.
- Minimum clinically significant improvement (MCSI) post intervention is 47.5 m.
- Better correlation with peak oxygen uptake than 6MWT but less well validated; also more cardiovascular risk.

6-minute walk test (6MWT)

- Patient walks quickly on a flat surface for 6 mins around a 30-m course.
- Allowed to stop and rest during the test; standard phrases of encouragement used.
- Normal estimates: 580 m (men), 500 m (women), significant improvement ≥ 54 m.
- Correlates well with functional scores of disability.

Cardiopulmonary exercise testing (CPX)

- Used to distinguish between respiratory and cardiac causes of breathlessness.
- Multiple parameters of lung function and cardiac function measured at rest.
- Repeated at incremental levels of exercise:
  - Cardiac function: ECG, BP, peak HR, and peak oxygen consumption.
  - Ventilatory function: tidal volume, expiratory capacity, spirometry.
  - Gas exchange efficiency: PaO_2, alveolar–arterial (A–a) gradient, oxygen saturations.

Respiratory muscle assessment

Diaphragm assessment

- Measure sitting or standing VC then repeat with patient lying supine:
  - Fall in VC <10%: probably normal.
  - Fall in VC 10–20%: suggests diaphragmatic weakness.
  - Fall in VC >20%: significant weakness or paralysis.
- Obesity causes resistance to diaphragm movement and may result in fall in supine VC without focal pathology.

Inspiratory muscle assessment

- Sniff test: measure negative pressure generated at the nose when sniffing:
  - Indication of inspiratory muscle strength.
- Transdiaphragmatic pressure measurement:
  - Balloons placed in oesophagus above and below diaphragm.
  - Measurement of diaphragmatic function.
- Phrenic nerve stimulation: using high-intensity magnets or electrical stimulation:
  - Passive assessment of diaphragmatic function.

Chapter 16

RESPIRATORY SCORING SYSTEMS AND STATISTICS

Respiratory scoring systems

Health status

- St Georges Respiratory Questionnaire:
  - ◆ Validated in patients with airway obstruction and bronchiectasis.
  - ◆ 50-item questionnaire assessing 3 domains: symptoms, activity, and impacts (psychosocial).
  - ◆ A change in score ≥4 units is considered significant.
  - ◆ Correlates with 6MWT and FEV_1.

Breathlessness

- BORG Scale:
  - ◆ Modified version rates perceived exertion from 0–10.
  - ◆ Patients with modified Borg score >0 are 3–5 times more likely to have impaired lung function.
- MRC dyspnoea score:

Table 16.1 MRC diapason score

Grade	Degree of breathlessness on activity
1	Not troubled by breathlessness except on strenuous exercise
2	Short of breath when hurrying or walking up a slight hill
3	Walks slower than contemporaries on level ground or has to stop for breath when walking at own pace
4	Stops for breath after walking 100 m or after a few minutes on level ground
5	Too breathless to leave the house or breathless on dressing/undressing

Performance status

- Karnofsky score:
  - ◆ Score from 0–100 where 0 is death and 100 is 'perfect' health.
- WHO/ECOG score.

Disease specific

Asthma

- Royal College of Physicians '3 questions':
  - ◆ In the last month/week have you had difficulty sleeping due to your asthma?
  - ◆ Have you had your usual asthma symptoms during the day?
  - ◆ Has your asthma interfered with your usual daily activities?
  - ◆ Interpretation:
    - ▪ One 'yes'—medium morbidity; ≥ 2 'yes' answers—high morbidity.

Table 16.2 WHO/ECOG performance score

Grade	
0	Fully active, no restrictions on activities.
1	Unable to do strenuous activities, but able to carry out light housework and sedentary activities.
2	Able to walk and manage self-care, but unable to work. Out of bed >50% of waking hours
3	Confined to bed or a chair >50% of waking hours. Capable of limited self-care.
4	Disabled. Totally confined to a bed or chair. Unable to self-care at all. Too breathless to leave the house or breathless on dressing/undressing
5	Dead

COPD

- BODE Index:
  - A 10-point scale calculated for 4 domains: body mass index, degree of airflow obstruction (FEV_1), dyspnoea (Modified MRC score), exercise capacity (6MWT).
  - Higher total score correlates to greater risk of death (from any cause).

Heart failure

- NYHA functional classification of heart failure:

Table 16.3 NYHA heart failure score

Grade	Symptoms on activity
I	No limitations. Ordinary physical activity does not cause symptoms of fatigue, breathlessness, palpitations, or chest pain
II	Slight limitation of physical activity. Ordinary physical activity results in mild symptoms. Comfortable at rest
III	Marked limitation of physical activity. Less than ordinary physical activity (e.g. walking short distances) will lead to symptoms. Comfortable only at rest
IV	Severe limitation. Symptomatic even at rest. Mostly bedbound

Pneumonia

- CURB65: see Chapter 4: Pulmonary infection.
- Pneumonia severity index:
  - Used to stratify patients with CAP into 5 risk categories, based on demographics, comorbidities, examination, CXR, and laboratory results.
  - 30-day mortality up to 30% for patients in category V (high risk).

Pulmonary embolism

- Well's score for PE:
  - Used to determine pre-test probability of PE; complicated by multiple versions being available.
  - 7 risk factors allocated weighted scores.
  - Interpretation:
    - Total score <2.0: low probability of PE.
    - Total score 2–6: moderate probability of PE.
    - Total score >6: high probability of PE.

- Geneva score:
    - Similar performance to the Well's score; independent of clinician judgement.
    - For modified score, total ≤ 2 indicates PE unlikely.

Sleep

- Epworth sleepiness scale: see Chapter 10: Sleep disorders.
- Pittsburgh Sleep Quality Index:
    - Self-rated questionnaire based on a 1-month period.
    - Total score ≥5 indicates poor sleep quality.

Illness severity

- Lung injury score (Murray score):
    - Used to characterize the severity of lung injury.
    - Scores calculated for 4 domains: consolidation on CXR, hypoxaemia ($PaO_2:FiO_2$), PEEP, and respiratory compliance.
    - Interpretation:
        - Total score 0: no lung injury.
        - Total score 0.1–2.5: mild-to-moderate lung injury.
        - Total score > 2.5: severe lung injury (ARDS).
    - ARDS defined by the combination of bilateral pulmonary infiltrates, PCWP <18 mmHg and $PaO_2:FiO_2$ < 200 mmHg:
        - For acute lung injury: $PaO_2:FiO_2$ < 300 mmHg.
- Scores used to predict mortality in patients admitted to intensive care:
    - Acute physiology and chronic health evaluation (APACHE II/III).
    - Sequential organ failure assessment (SOFA).
    - Simplified acute physiology score (SAPS II).

Study design and statistics

Data types

- Categorical:
    - Binary: e.g. male/female.
    - Nominal: e.g. ethnic group (no order).
    - Ordinal: e.g. mild/moderate/severe COPD (ordered).
- Numerical: continuous/discrete.
- Paired/unpaired:
    - Whether or not a one-to-one relationship exists between values in 2 data sets.

Descriptive statistics

- Mean: sum of all observations divided by the total number of observations.
- Median: middle value when all observations are ranked in order.
- Mode: most frequent observation.
- Normal distribution:
    - Mean, median, and mode are equal.
    - Frequency distribution is symmetrical (bell shaped).
- Centile:
    - The value below which a given percentage of observations lie.

- ◆ The 50th centile is equivalent to the median.
- ◆ The 25th and 75th centiles are known as quartiles; the difference between these is the interquartile range.
- Standard deviation (SD): a measure of the scatter of values around the mean; the higher the value the greater the spread of data.
- Standard error of mean: a measure of how well the study sample reflects the true findings in the wider population.

Study design

- Study types:
  - ◆ Prospective/retrospective.
  - ◆ Cross sectional (single time point)/longitudinal (serial observations).
  - ◆ Observational/experimental.
- Observational studies:
  - ◆ Case–control: subjects with condition of interest are compared with subjects who do not have the condition but are otherwise similar:
    - ▪ Usually retrospective.
    - ▪ Quick, cheap, require fewer patients than cohort studies, can measure rare outcomes.
    - ▪ Suggest association but cannot demonstrate causality.
  - ◆ Cohort: exposed and unexposed subjects are observed over a given time period for the development of an outcome of interest:
    - ▪ Usually prospective.
    - ▪ Can measure multiple outcomes; demonstrate causality.
- Experimental studies:
  - ◆ Randomized controlled trials: subjects are randomly allocated to receive an intervention or no intervention/standard care:
    - ▪ Minimizes bias and spurious causality.
- Null hypothesis:
  - ◆ The assertion that there is no difference between observed groups.
- P value:
  - ◆ Probability of getting the results obtained, given the null hypothesis is true; conventional significance is taken as $p < 0.05$.
- Tests of difference:
  - ◆ Parametric: for normally distributed data:
    - ▪ T-test: continuous data, paired or unpaired; used to compare mean values for 2 independent groups or against hypothesized values.
    - ▪ Analysis of variance: continuous data; used to compare means for multiple groups.
  - ◆ Non-parametric: for data that is *not* normally distributed:
    - ▪ Mann–Whitney U test: discrete, unpaired data; compares the median values for 2 independent groups.
    - ▪ Wilcoxon signed rank test: discrete, paired data; the non-parametric analogue to the paired T-test.
    - ▪ Chi-square test: categorical data; used to test goodness of fit to a hypothesis or to determine the relationship between categorical variables.
    - ▪ Fisher's exact test: used instead of the chi-square test when 1 or more cells has an expected frequency of ≤ 5.

- Correlation:
  - Used to demonstrate the linear relationship between ≥2 normally distributed, continuous variables.
  - Correlation coefficient quantifies the degree of correlation:
    - Values from −1 to +1.
  - Spearman rank correlation used for non-normally distributed variables.
- Regression:
  - Simple *linear* regression is used to demonstrate relationship between a continuous, independent (predictor) variable and a continuous, dependent (outcome) variable.
  - In simple *logistic* regression a continuous, independent variable is measured against a dichotomous dependent variable.
  - Multiple regression involves ≥1 independent variable.

Population statistics

- Incidence: the number of new cases detected over a given time period in the population at risk.
- Prevalence: the number of existing cases at a single time point.
- Absolute risk: the rate of occurrence; comparable to incidence.
- Relative risk: the proportion of cases in exposed vs. non-exposed individuals.

Screening tests

- Sensitivity: the proportion of positive results correctly identified by the test.
- Specificity: the proportion of negative results correctly identified by the test.
- Positive predictive value: the proportion of patients with positive results that are correctly diagnosed.
- Negative predictive value: the proportion of patients with negative results that are correctly diagnosed.

1. D. *Mycoplasma*, *Chlamydia*, and (variably) *Leigonella* are considered atypical pathogens in pneumonia. All may cause a 'flu like illness followed by a dry cough. Features of *Mycoplasma* include autoimmune haemolytic anaemia (secondary to cold agglutinins), thrombocytopenia, SIADH, erythema multiforme (target lesions on limbs and trunk), and Stevens–Johnson syndrome (rash plus mucosal involvement). Guillain–Barré syndrome is also described.

2. C. The combination of restrictive spirometry with reduced lung volumes and transfer factor suggest a pulmonary parenchymal pathology. In this scenario, RA-ILD is the most likely diagnosis. ILD is the most common pulmonary manifestation of RA and may onset before joint symptoms. Prevalence is up to 40% with peak age 50–60 years, males > females. RA-associated lung disease may also manifest as rheumatoid nodules (solitary or multiple, can cavitate), pleural effusions (exudative, pH <7.2, glucose <1.6, LDH >700, raised cholesterol), pneumothoraces, and rarely bronchiectasis and bronchiolitis obliterans. RA-ILD may mimic IPF (UIP) or NSIP. Treatment with anti-inflammatory agents (prednisone) and immunomodulators (azathioprine/cyclophosphamide) is recommended. Avoid anti-TNF agents (cause accelerated death from ILD) and methotrexate. Caplan's syndrome, the combination of pneumoconiosis with rheumatoid factor positivity, is associated with exposure to mining dust. Shrinking lung syndrome is associated with SLE, the features being reduced lung volumes due to diaphragmatic weakness but preserved KCO. Pulmonary arterial hypertension typically manifests as an isolated reduction in TLCO/KCO.

3. B. Chronic eosinophilic pneumonia consists of chronic fever, cough, sweats, and weight loss. It is most common in middle-aged women. It is not an infective process but an exaggerated eosinophilic response. Serum eosinophil levels are not grossly elevated but sputum/BAL levels are raised. CXR typically shows an inverse pulmonary oedema pattern. TB is often in the differential. Tropical pulmonary eosinophilia is caused by filarial worms. Loeffler's syndrome is either asymptomatic or gives a brief respiratory illness with larvae found in the sputum. She has no history of wheeze or asthma to fit with Churg–Strauss syndrome. Acute pulmonary eosinophilia is a diagnosis of exclusion with a short history of fever and hypoxia.

4. E. This woman has periodic limb movement disorder (PLMD). Diagnosis requires typical limb movements on polysomnography (i.e. repetitive, 0.5–5 seconds duration, separated by an interval of 5–90 seconds, measured at tibialis anterior), ≥5 periodic limb movements per hour of sleep, clinical evidence of sleep disturbance, and no alternative cause for the movement disorder/sleep disturbance. The condition is more prevalent with age. Sex distribution is equal. Benzodiazepines and dopamine agonists are often used to treat PLMD. Non-ergot dopamine agonists, pramipexole and ropinirole, cause fewer side effects and are considered first line. If PMLD is associated with restless leg syndrome, gabapentin and opioids/opioid agonists may also be beneficial. Antidepressants, antipsychotic agents, dopamine antagonists (e.g. metoclopramide), and sedating antihistamines may exacerbate restless leg symptoms, as may caffeine, nicotine, and alcohol. Modafinil (a CNS stimulant) and CPAP are treatments for OSA. Daytime somnolence in this case results from periodic limb movements causing partial/total arousal from sleep, not from OSA.

5. E. This patient has a 1.8-cm primary pneumothorax. Even though this is small, he is breathless so requires intervention.

6. A. All patients commenced on non-invasive ventilation (NIV) need a treatment failure plan clearly documented in the medical notes. This must include a decision about resuscitation and escalation of care. Even in obese patients the BIPAP settings should start as low as possible (IPAP 10 cmH$_2$O and EPAP 5 cmH$_2$O) and the IPAP then rapidly increased. This improves patient comfort and tolerance of NIV. A nasal BIPAP mask may be preferred once the patient is stable, but in the first 24 hours a full face mask is recommended. A starting pH of <7.26 does not preclude NIV but does increase the risk of failure. Oxygen saturations should be maintained between 89–92%.

7. E. T-tests are used to compare a single, continuous, variable across two groups, when the data is parametric and follows a normal distribution. The paired T-test is used when the two groups are matched (e.g. pre/post intervention or case–control). The unpaired T-test is used when the groups are not matched. The chi-square test is used to compare categorical variables (e.g. ethnicity, hair colour). The Mann–Whitney U test is used to compare discrete variables (e.g. 5-point rating scale), when data is non-parametric. The correlation coefficient is used to compare the relationship between two continuous variables. Logistic regression compares a continuous, independent variable against a dichotomous, dependent (outcome) variable.

8. E. This CT shows a lesion in the anterior mediastinum (anterior to the pericardium) which appears as a well-defined, oval soft tissue mass. The most common anterior mediastinal masses are thymomas. These occur equally in males and females, and usually present from age 30–50 years. 50% of patients with thymoma have myasthenia gravis and 15% of patients with myasthenia have thymoma. Other paraneoplastic syndromes occurring with thymoma include red cell aplasia, and hypogammaglobulinaemia.

Mediastinal teratomas are usually larger in size than thymomas. They are cystic in nature and may contain skin, hair, sweat glands, sebaceous material, bone, or tooth-like structures, visible on CT. Radiological features of thyroid goitre are well-defined borders, high attenuation in the absence of intravenous contrast, punctate calcification, and early prolonged enhancement after contrast, ± tracheal displacement. Bronchogenic cysts are congenital anomalies of foregut origin which appear as sharply marginated masses of low attenuation.

9. E. According to the 7th edition of the TNM classification of lung cancer, this woman has stage IIIA (T3 N1 M0) disease and her WHO performance status is 1. According to the BTS, all patients with T1a–3 N0–1 M0 disease should be considered for radical treatment. Since she is unfit for surgery, which is considered first line, she should be offered radical radiotherapy. Patients with locally advanced (stage II/III) disease should be considered for combined chemoradiotherapy. Chemotherapy alone has no curative effect and is not appropriate in this patient. Palliative radiotherapy is typically reserved for symptom control in patients with stage IV disease and impaired performance status.

10. B. This patient has acute severe asthma which has failed to respond to nebulized bronchodilators and steroids. A single dose of intravenous magnesium (1.2–2.0 g) is the appropriate management option. Intravenous salbutamol and theophylline are not routinely recommended for the treatment of acute asthma. NIV has not been shown to be beneficial in acute asthma and patients requiring ventilatory support should be referred for consideration of intubation.

Whilst the most common acid–base abnormality in acute asthma is respiratory alkalosis, metabolic acidosis occurs in over 28% of patients due to lactic acidosis. The pathogenesis is thought to relate to tissue hypoxia but $\beta2$ agonists may have a contributory effect. Theophylline is also recognized to cause lactic acidosis and metabolic acidosis in a patient on oral theophylline should raise the suspicion of toxicity.

11. E. This CT demonstrates ground-glass attenuation with peripheral reticulation and traction bronchiectasis but minimal honeycombing. The distribution is diffuse but there is relative sparing of the subpleural areas. These features are in keeping with NSIP, which is the most common pulmonary manifestation of connective tissue disease. By contrast, IPF, of which UIP is the histological pattern, typically demonstrates a patchy, peripheral, basal distribution with a predominance of honeycomb fibrosis and architectural distortion with traction bronchiectasis and minimal ground-glass change. Temporal and spatial heterogeneity in IPF results in areas of pathology interspersed with normal lung. Hypersensitivity pneumonitis manifests as ill-defined centrilobular nodules or as a mosaic pattern sparing the lung bases but end-stage disease may be indistinguishable from IPF. The presence of coexistent pleural plaques help to identify asbestosis. Sarcoidosis manifests as bilateral, symmetrical hilar and mediastinal lymphadenopathy with interlobular septal thickening/beading and centrilobular nodules, predominantly affecting the upper lobes. Hypersensitivity pneumonitis and sarcoidosis are less common in smokers.

12. B. The spirometry shows an obstructive pattern and the flow volume loop shows evidence of flattening on both the inspiratory and expiratory curves confirming fixed upper airway obstruction. This can be due to postintubation stenosis (or post-tracheostomy stenosis), goitres, and upper airway tumours. Given her history, a postintubation stenosis is the most likely pathology. Tracheomalacia produces variable intrathoracic airway obstruction with a normal inspiratory curve but flattened expiratory curve on flow volume loop. Vocal cord paralysis produces variable extrathoracic obstruction and therefore a flattened inspiratory curve but normal expiratory curve on flow volume loop. Postventilation fibrosis is a parenchymal pathology and produces restrictive spirometry. A chest wall deformity would normally show restrictive spirometry.

13. A. The CT shows the halo sign with ground-glass opacity surrounding a pulmonary nodule or mass. The reversed halo sign is a focal rounded area of ground-glass opacity surrounded by a crescent or complete ring of consolidation. Both the halo sign and the reversed halo sign are highly suggestive of fungal infection in an immunocompromised patient. The differential diagnosis for this CT finding in an immunocompromised patient includes invasive/semi-invasive fungal disease, metastases with surrounding inflammation, or occasionally septic emboli and haemorrhage. The halo of ground-glass attenuation in this CT pathologically represents non-haemorrhagic inflammatory processes.

14. E. The findings in this patient are consistent with respiratory bronchiolitis-interstitial lung disease (RB-ILD), rather than desquamative interstitial pneumonia, in which pigmented macrophages are evenly dispersed within alveolar spaces. Initial management in all cases is smoking cessation, which results in disease stabilization or improvement in up to two-thirds of patients. Inhaled steroids may be indicated as part of therapy for concurrent COPD but are not a recognized treatment for RB-ILD. In patients who fail to improve or deteriorate in the 3 months after smoking cessation, oral prednisolone is indicated (1 mg/kg, tapered after 1 month, duration of therapy typically 1 year), although the benefits are controversial. Azathioprine may be used as a steroid-sparing agent in patients responsive to prednisolone.

15. B. This patient has a typical presentation of simple pulmonary eosinophilia (Loeffler's syndrome) which is caused by *Ascaris lumbricoides, Strongyloides*, and other helminths. Her travel history is not relevant as these helminths are found worldwide. If symptomatic, treatment is with an antihelminth agent such as mebendazole.

16. A. Based on his history and polysomnography results this patient has moderate OSA. Falling asleep at the wheel is a criminal offence and may lead to imprisonment. The patient is responsible for informing the DVLA of his diagnosis but the consulting physician must ensure he receives this information verbally, in writing, and copied to his GP. Patients with OSA can retain a group 1 (car/motorcycle) licence; they should not drive if they have symptoms of excessive sleepiness during waking hours but can restart driving as soon as their symptoms are controlled on therapy. Patients with a group 2 licence should cease driving until satisfactory symptom control is achieved *and* confirmed by a specialist. Licensing reviews will be carried out regularly, usually annually.

17. C. Following spontaneous pneumothorax the current BTS guidelines suggest that it is safe to fly once CXR shows complete resolution but recommend waiting for at least 7 days. There is no need for pleurodesis after a first episode of pneumothorax; however, it may reduce risk of recurrence and patients who have had a surgical pleurodesis can fly once they have recovered from surgery. Following traumatic pneumothorax a period of 2 weeks after complete CXR resolution is recommended.

18. D. A low-volume, high-frequency, high PEEP strategy has been shown to reduce the incidence of ventilator-induced lung damage and ARDS. On this basis, the ideal TV for this woman is between 4–6 ml/kg (360–480 ml) so 400 ml is the closest. Increasing her total ventilation, or minute volume (MV), will decrease her pCO_2 and help to correct her acidosis. You can do this by either increasing her RR or TV. The TV should not be increased above 6 ml/kg as above. If her RR increases too far (>35 bpm) the dead space ventilation increases so making her ventilation less effective. She is hypoxic with pO_2 6.2. To improve her oxygenation you can either increase the FiO_2 (not possible in this case) or increase the PEEP. Mechanically ventilated patients will often require a PEEP of 10–15 cm to maintain adequate oxygenation.

19. D. LVRS aims to remove 20–30% of lung volume in order to improve airflow, diaphragm and chest wall mechanics and alveolar gas exchange in the remaining portion of the lung. It may be used as an alternative to transplantation in severe COPD. Indications for LVRS (derived from the National Emphysema Treatment Trial) are age <75 years, severe dyspnoea despite maximal medical therapy, FEV_1 <45% predicted, TLCO >20% predicted, lung volumes indicative of gas trapping (RV >150% predicted, TLC >100% predicted, increased RV:TLC ratio), heterogeneously distributed emphysema on CT, 6MWT >140 m, and abstinence from smoking for ≥6 months. Contraindications are comorbid illness, extremes of BMI, poor rehabilitation potential, thoracic deformity, previous thoracic surgery, minimal or homogeneously distributed emphysema on CT (particularly if FEV_1 <20% predicted), giant bullae (bullectomy preferable), interstitial lung disease, pulmonary nodules, and pulmonary hypertension. LVRS appears most beneficial in patients with upper lobe disease. Patients with A1AT deficiency appear to derive less benefit.

20. B. Systemic steroids are the mainstay of therapy for Churg–Strauss. In patients with evidence of systemic vasculitis, prednisolone is commenced at 1 mg/kg/day for remission-induction, and then tapered over a period of 12 months. In multisystem or life-threatening disease, IV methylprednisolone (1 g three times a day) is given for 3 days, followed by standard prednisolone therapy. Premature withdrawal of treatment can result in recurrence. Patients with extrapulmonary involvement, particularly cardiac and central nervous system, usually require additional immunosuppression. Cyclophosphamide (2 mg/kg/day) is used in combination with steroids for patients with severe, multiorgan disease. Once remission is induced with cyclophosphamide and steroid therapy, patients are switched to maintenance therapy with azathioprine or methotrexate, in combination with a tapering dose of steroids.

21. B. In patients with symptomatic malignant effusions, intervention is indicated. Therapeutic aspiration may provide symptomatic relief but the high rate of effusion recurrence means aspiration is not recommended in patients with a life expectancy >1 month. In patients other than those with a very short life expectancy, small bore (10–14 F) intercostal drain insertion followed by pleurodesis is the preferred management. Intrapleural fibrinolytics are recommended for symptomatic multiloculated effusions resistant to drainage. Where there is incomplete apposition of the pleura following drainage i.e. 'trapped lung', pleurodesis may still be attempted (if >50% apposition) or an indwelling catheter sited. Talc is the most effective agent for pleurodesis; bleomycin is an alternative. In patients with good performance status, thorascopic drainage and talc poudrage is recommended.

22. A. This CXR demonstrates an azygous fissure running horizontally in the right upper zone. This is a congenital malformation which occurs in 1–2% of individuals. Anomalous passage of the azygous vein creates an anatomically separated portion of the upper lobe, which has no bronchi or vasculature of its own (i.e. not a true or accessory lobe). There is no associated morbidity although it may lead to technical problems during bronchoscopy/thoracoscopy. The finding of a preserved lung volume, a non-displaced horizontal fissure, and the absence of a triangular apical opacity goes against right upper lobe collapse in this case. Pulmonary agenesis, in which a lobe (or entire lung), its bronchi, and vessels fail to develop, mimics lobar collapse or lobectomy. Bronchopulmonary sequestration occurs when there is a non-functioning mass of lung tissue that lacks normal communication with the tracheobronchial tree and receives its arterial blood supply from the systemic circulation. Sequestered tissue typically appears as a dense mass on CXR but recurrent infection may lead to cystic change. Intrapulmonary bronchogenic cysts appear well demarcated and often contain fluid/mucus.

23. A. This is a 2×2 contingency table, used to record the relationship between two categorical variables. The chi-square test is appropriate for the analysis of this type of data. Fisher's exact test is also used to analyse contingency tables but where sample sizes are small. The T-test is used to compare two continuous variables and requires parametric data. QALY analysis is used for economic modelling and provides cost–benefit data for medical interventions. Kaplan–Meier analysis is widely used to estimate survival function but requires survival data from multiple time points, usually over a prolonged period.

24. C. Whole-body plethysmography measures communicating and non-communicating lung volumes and therefore will give a TLC that includes all bullous disease. Helium dilution TLC measurement can only measure communicating lung volume and can also be falsely reduced by failure of the helium to diffuse into the smaller peripheral (and sometimes obstructed) airways. TLCO may be reduced in bullous disease. Cardiopulmonary exercise testing is used to distinguish between cardiac and respiratory causes of breathlessness and is not helpful here.

25. B. Pneumoconiosis is considered to have no malignant potential. Simple pneumoconiosis is non-progressive once exposure ceases. In PMF there is slowly progressive coalescence of pulmonary nodules to form large upper zone opacities (>10-mm diameter) with fibrosis and cavitation in advanced disease or in the context of mycobacterial superinfection. Patients with PMF may seek compensation under the Workers' Compensation Act. Nodules in Caplan's syndrome are considered to be benign. The frequency of symptomatic obstructive lung disease is higher in all coal miners, irrespective of smoking history.

26. A. HPS is the combination of liver disease, pulmonary vascular dilatation (± pleural and pulmonary arteriovenous malformation), and hypoxaemia. Platypnoea (worsening dyspnoea on sitting up from a supine position) and orthodexia (a decrease in pO_2 ≥0.5 kPa or in oxygen saturation ≥5% on moving from supine to upright) are seen in up to 88% of patients with HPS. Contrast-enhanced transthoracic echocardiography with agitated saline (microbubbles ≥10 μm) is the most practical method to detect pulmonary vascular dilatation. Bubble echo is more sensitive and less invasive than injection of radiolabelled (technetium-99) macroaggregated albumin for lung scanning. Pulmonary angiography is only indicated in patients with severe hypoxemia poorly responsive to oxygen therapy and when there is a high likelihood (based on CT chest) of direct arteriovenous communications that may be amenable to embolization. Right heart catheterization is used to diagnose porto-pulmonary hypertension, features of which are vasoconstriction, endothelial and smooth muscle proliferation, thrombosis, and arteriopathy. Reduced TLCO is the only consistent pulmonary function test abnormality in patients with HPS; however, reduced TLCO is not specific to the condition.

27. E. All of the ethical principles are relevant to this case. If a patient has the capacity to make informed choices regarding treatment options, their autonomy should be respected. In patients who lack capacity, advance directives may be used as documentation of their wishes. This patient's note does not meet the criteria for a valid advance directive and is therefore not legally binding. Furthermore, doctors are not legally obliged to provide treatment they feel is inappropriate. Beneficence is the process of balancing the benefits of treatment against the risks whilst non-maleficence is the avoidance of causing harm. Intensive care which may prolong duration of life at the expense of quality may be considered detrimental in this case. Justice relates to the equitable distribution of resources. Intensive care for this patient may not to be cost-effective and may impact upon the availability of treatment for others.

28. A. Many asthmatics dive safely but those with exercise-induced asthma, recent exacerbation, or use of reliever medication in the preceding 48 hours should not dive. Previous traumatic pneumothorax is not a contraindication but a CT chest should be performed to ensure complete resolution before diving is approved. Spontaneous pneumothorax is of greater concern and is more likely to recur. Treatment with bilateral surgical pleurodesis or pleurectomy significantly reduces this risk; however, there is some concern about cerebral air embolism and pneumomediastinum. Previous tuberculosis is not a contraindication but may require CXR/CT scanning to ensure no bullae are present. Sinusitis may cause problems with pressure equalizing on descent and ascent, but if well controlled is not an independent contraindication.

29. E. This is a young, underweight woman with a history shortness of breath and who has taken appetite suppressants. Her ventilatory function is normal, but with reduced TLCO and KCO. Cardiopulmonary exercise testing helps to distinguish between cardiac and respiratory origin of breathlessness but would not be particularly helpful here. Anaemia might explain the reduced transfer factors but a more worrying diagnosis is pulmonary hypertension secondary to use of fenfluramine (an appetite suppressant). This would be confirmed on right heart catheterization.

A HRCT would help diagnose interstitial lung disease but she has no other signs to support this and her RV and TLC are normal. A significantly low TLCO and KCO should not be ignored in a woman with this history.

30. B. Sensitivity is a measure of the proportion of patients with disease, correctly identified by the test. Specificity is a measure of the proportion of patients without disease, correctly identified by the test. The positive predictive value of a test is the proportion of patients with a positive test result that are correctly diagnosed. Similarly, the negative predictive value is the proportion of patients with a negative test result who have no disease. Absolute risk describes the actual difference in outcome occurrence in different exposure groups. Relative risk describes the ratio of outcome occurrence in exposed versus non-exposed groups. Odds ratio is a measure of relative risk, defined as the ratio of the odds of exposure in cases to the odds of exposure in controls.

31. D. The CT shows cystic lung disease, evidenced by focal regions of low attenuation with well-defined walls. Cysts are typically thin walled (<2 mm), air or fluid filled. Non-infective causes include LCH, LAM, tuberous sclerosis, lymphoid interstitial pneumonia, and IPF. Infective causes include *Pneumocystis jiroveci* pneumonia and *Staphylococcus*. The radiological pattern in this case suggests LAM, with round cysts of <2-cm diameter diffusely distributed throughout the entire lungs.

In LCH, cysts are typically associated with nodules, have irregular, bizarre shapes, and are randomly distributed throughout the upper and middle lungs, sparing the bases. Cysts in IPF are subpleural with thick fibrous walls and a basilar predominance. Blebs are intrapleural. Scans for catamenial pneumothorax are often negative unless they are obtained during menses but may show small cavities, nodules, or ground-glass infiltrates suggestive of local haemorrhage. Emphysema may mimic cystic lung disease; however, emphysematous airspaces have no discernible walls and occasional central vessels. Bronchiectatic cysts display the signet ring sign due to an accompanying artery in their wall.

32. E. All patients about to start on anti-TNF therapy or renal replacement therapy should be screened for active and latent TB infection. TST is difficult to interpret in an adult patient on steroids from a high-risk area and an IGRA does not differentiate between active and latent disease. She is from a high-risk country and has evidence of previous TB infection on her CXR with no history of treatment. She has no symptoms suggestive of active TB so she should be treated for latent TB infection on the basis of her CXR.

33. E. This woman is in the early stages of motor neurone disease as suggested by the change in speech and progressive respiratory muscle weakness shown by a restrictive pattern on PFT with normal transfer factor. There is a significant fall in VC on lying down which suggests diaphragmatic weakness or paralysis. Guillain–Barré usually occurs following an acute illness and consists of an ascending neuropathy which affects the respiratory muscles and causes respiratory failure but this would be an unusual initial presentation. IPF and hypersensitivity pneumonitis would explain the restrictive lung function, but not the fall in vital capacity when lying down. Obese patients often have restrictive spirometry with reduced TLCO but KCO should be normal (not given here). Obesity can also cause a fall in VC when lying but a drop of 22% is pathological and obesity would not explain her change in speech.

34. A. This man has stage IA disease (T1b N0 M0) and provided there are no medical contraindications and he has adequate lung function, he should be considered a candidate for surgical resection. Surgery should aim to conserve lung volume by non-anatomical resection or lobectomy in preference to pneumonectomy. Neither chemotherapy nor radiotherapy is recommended preoperatively. Postoperative management depends on whether there is complete resection of the tumour. If the tumour is not completely resected, the patient should be offered radiotherapy (adjuvant, not radical) to improve local disease control. If resection is complete, adjuvant chemotherapy may be offered following discussion of the risks and benefits. There is no role for postoperative combined chemoradiotherapy. Cranial irradiation is reserved for patients with small cell lung cancer whose disease is responsive to treatment.

35. B. Phenotypically and pathologically, there is an overlap between asthma and COPD, which can make it difficult to differentiate the two conditions. Asthma is characterized by episodic, reversible airway obstruction and airway hyper-responsiveness. With time this reversibility may become incomplete. COPD is characterized by fixed airflow obstruction and is associated with parenchymal features inducing the loss of lung elastic recoil (increased compliance), resting and dynamic lung hyperinflation. Both chemically-induced (methacholine/histamine) and exercise-induced hyper-responsiveness are defining characteristics of asthma. Bronchodilator reversibility is greater in asthma than COPD and asthmatics are more likely to demonstrate an improvement in FEV1 following a 2-week trial of oral prednisolone. Diffusing capacity is typically normal or increased in asthma and decreased in COPD. CT changes are poor discriminators between asthma and COPD, particularly in asthmatics who smoke.

36. E. Pulmonary hypertension (PH) is a recognized complication of obstructive sleep apnoea, particularly when it is combined with obesity hypoventilation syndrome or other causes of hypoxaemia. Prevalence of PH in OSA is 15–20%. PH is defined by a mPAP ≥25 mmHg at rest. PH resulting from causes other than left-sided cardiac lesions and pulmonary vein compression is associated with a PCWP <15 mmHg. Features on ECHO include paradoxical bulging of the septum into the left ventricle and right ventricular (RV) hypertrophy, progressing to RV dilation and hypokinesis, right atrial dilation, and tricuspid regurgitation. Obesity typically results in a restrictive defect on pulmonary function testing; transfer factor is reduced in concurrent PH. Positive airway pressure therapy reduces pulmonary arterial systolic pressure but the reduction is modest and evidence of improved patient outcomes is limited.

37. B. This is a hamartoma, the CT features of which are a solitary, round, smooth mass containing fat and 'popcorn' calcification, typically peripheral in location (although 10% are endobronchial). Hamartomas are comprised of tissues normally found in the lung but in abnormal quantities or arrangements. They are the most common benign lung mass and account for around 8% of all solitary pulmonary nodules. Prevalence peaks in the 5th and 6th decade and there is a male to female ratio of 3:1. Calcification suggests benign disease. Wegener's granulomatosis typically presents with multiple basal nodules of varying sizes, which frequently cavitate. Tuberculomas are most commonly found in the apical or posterior segments of the upper lobes or the superior segments of the lower lobes. These manifest as round/oval lesions often with calcification, adjacent tree-in-bud lesions, or small, discrete shadows in the immediate vicinity ('satellite' lesions).

38. C. Patients with pneumothoraces and a persistent air leak or failure of lung expansion should be considered for early referral to the thoracic surgeons. Referral at 48 hours is currently recommended for secondary pneumothorax and 3–5 days for primary pneumothorax. Suction should be considered after 48 hours if there is evidence of ongoing leak or incomplete resolution. Continuous high-volume, low-pressure suction is recommended with pressure between −10 to −20 cmH₂O.

39. A. At first, isolation it is important to attempt eradication of *Pseudomonas*, normally using both ciprofloxacin and a nebulized antipseudomonal (e.g. colomycin). Successful eradication should be confirmed with at least two negative sputum cultures. Chronic colonization with *Pseudomonas* can be managed with antibiotic nebulizers to reduce bacterial load. The patient should be isolated from patients without *Pseudomonas* and also from those with mucoid *Pseudomonas* which carries a worse prognosis.

40. D. This HIV positive patient has a prolonged history of cough and shortness of breath. This would fit with many diagnoses, but the normal CXR associated with hypoxia makes TB less likely. Although viral pneumonia/pneumonitis is possible and could cause exercise desaturation the most likely cause is PCP. Urgent HRCT and bronchoscopy are both valuable investigations, but starting treatment is the most important step. Bronchoscopy samples remain positive for PCP for up to 5 days following treatment. It is important to add steroids as he is hypoxic.

41. E. Her CXR demonstrates prominence of the left hilar vasculature (proximal dilatation) and distal oligaemia due to vasoconstriction (Westermark's sign). These features are consistent with acute thromboembolism. Westermark's sign is seen in 2% of cases. Other CXR changes include hemidiaphragm elevation, pleural effusion, discoid atelectasis (subsegmental, plate-like), and pulmonary infiltrates (basal, wedge shaped, abutting the pleural surface, known as Hampton's hump; may be confused with infection). Cardiomegaly is commonly seen on CXR but does not correlate with right ventricular hypokinesis by ECHO. PH manifests as bilateral enlargement of the central pulmonary arteries with attenuation of peripheral vessels and bilateral oligaemia, ± right ventricular enlargement and right atrial dilatation (prominent right heart border). Diagnosis can only be confirmed by right heart catheterization. Fat embolism typically occurs following lower limb or pelvic fracture. Features are dyspnoea, confusion, petechial rash, and hypocalcaemia. CXR demonstrates a pulmonary oedema-like image.

42. D. The risk of death from TB is higher in HIV positive patients and treatment for both should be started promptly; however, the complex drug interactions, side effects, and pill burden mean it is not recommended to commence TB treatment and HAART simultaneously. The current WHO guidelines recommend starting TB treatment as soon as possible, followed by HAART at 2 weeks (or at least within 8 weeks). HAART-mediated immune reconstitution may cause a paradoxical deterioration in a patient established on TB treatment. HAART should be started in all HIV positive patients with TB, regardless of CD4 count.

43. D. This CT scan demonstrates diffuse, ground-glass opacification which alone is non-specific but in the context of the history is suggestive of diffuse alveolar haemorrhage (DAH). DAH is a rare yet serious complication of a variety of disorders. Three histological patterns are recognized—pulmonary capillaritis, bland pulmonary haemorrhage (without alveolar inflammation, e.g. coagulopathy), and diffuse alveolar damage (associated with ARDS). Most cases of DAH are caused by pulmonary capillaritis associated with autoimmune disease such as Wegener's, anti-glomerular basement membrane (GBM) disease, and SLE. Pulmonary renal syndromes may result in concurrent alveolar haemorrhage and focal segmental glomerulonephritis. Idiopathic pulmonary haemosiderosis is primarily seen in younger patients and is established by lung biopsy which demonstrates bland pulmonary haemorrhage without immune complexes.

TLCO is a sensitive marker for DAH. Treatment should be targeted to the underlying disease but prompt immunosuppression (steroids ± cyclophosphamide) is indicated for DAH associated with vasculitis, connective tissue disease, and anti-GBM disease. Plasma exchange is commonly used to treat anti-GBM disease.

44. B. There are many areas in which swine 'flu is endemic in pig populations. There are also some ongoing outbreaks of H1N1 influenza during the 'flu season. Although in the majority of patients the H1N1 virus is relatively mild, those with multiple comorbidities and pregnant women are most at risk. Pregnant women are at increased risk of hospitalization, admission to ICU and death with H1N1. Infection is also associated with increased neonatal morbidity and mortality. Early treatment (<48 hours) offers some protection. The DOH and WHO recommend vaccination particularly for healthcare workers and pregnant women.

45. E. In this scenario, the null hypothesis would assert that there is no difference in efficacy between the new medication and the placebo. A statistical test can either reject (prove false) or fail to reject (fail to prove false) a null hypothesis, but can never prove it true. A type I error, also known as a false positive, occurs when a statistical test rejects a true null hypothesis. A type II error, also known as a false negative, occurs when the test fails to reject a false null hypothesis. The most common cause of a type II error is small sample size, leading to an underpowered study.

46. A. This CT demonstrates diffuse pleural thickening (DPT), with a contiguous irregular pleural peel, fibrous strands (crow's feet), parenchymal bands, and ipsilateral volume loss. DPT characteristically affects the visceral pleura, extending >8 cm cranio-caudally and involving >5 cm of the chest wall in cross section, with a thickness >3 mm. The costophrenic angles are often involved. CT features that may be helpful in distinguishing malignant (i.e. mesothelioma, metastatic disease) from benign pleural disease include circumferential thickening, nodular thickening, thickness >1 cm, and involvement of the mediastinal pleura. Calcification suggests a benign process. Pleural plaques appear as discrete areas of pleural thickening, often with calcification, which preferentially involve the parietal pleura adjacent to ribs 6–9 and the diaphragm. Shrinking pleuritis is another name for rounded atelectasis in which retractile visceral pleural fibrosis creates a comet-tail appearance at the basal lung periphery with in-drawing of vascular components. Ankylosing spondylitis causes pleuro-pulmonary disease in <2% of patients, most commonly in the form of chest wall restriction and upper lobe interstitial disease.

47. C. CF is the third most common indication for lung transplantation and survival rates are higher than for other conditions. Colonization with resistant *Pseudomonas*, MRSA, *Stenotrophomonas*, and *Aspergillus* is not known to affect outcome and is not a contraindication to transplantation. *Burkholderia cepacia* colonization (particularly genomovar III) is associated with increased mortality post-transplant and is a relative contraindication. Low BMI is not considered a contraindication; however, pretransplant obesity is a significant risk for mortality and BMI >30 kg/m^2 is a relative contraindication. Pleurodesis and pleurectomy increase the technical difficulty of extracting the native lung but should not preclude transplantation.

Exacerbation of CF requiring invasive ventilation indicates increasing disease severity and is an indication for transplant assessment. Patients requiring ongoing invasive ventilation should only be considered if they have been evaluated and listed before the onset of ventilatory assistance, they have been informed that worsening of their clinical situation after intubation may eventually contraindicate transplantation, they have no other significant organ dysfunction, and they agree to proceed to intubation.

48. A. For atypical mycobacterium a minimum of two positive cultures are required to confirm diagnosis before treatment. From sterile sites (ascites, pleural fluid) then one positive culture is sufficient in a patient with consistent physical signs and/or symptoms. A confirmed MAI diagnosis will normally require 24 months of rifampicin and ethambutol.

49. C. This is a case of lymphangitis carcinomatosis, occurring due to infiltration and obstruction of pulmonary lymphatic channels by tumour. Tumours which metastasize via the lymphatics include breast, lung, colon, stomach, pancreas, thyroid, cervix, prostate, and larynx. 80% are adenocarcinomas. There is rapid onset and progression of symptoms, which often precede CXR changes. Appearances on CXR are non-specific but include diffuse reticulonodular opacification, septal lines, peribronchial cuffing, pleural effusions, and mediastinal/hilar lymphadenopathy. On CT chest, thickening of the interlobular septae and bronchovascular structures create the appearance of polygonal arcades with central dots.

Lymphangitis is often asymmetrically distributed, which is useful in distinguishing it from pulmonary oedema. In sarcoidosis and lymphoma reticular change tends to progress from the perihilar region to the periphery whilst lymphangitis has a more diffuse distribution. Bronchoalveolar cell carcinoma may be present as a solitary nodule or as an infiltrative lesion resembling pneumonia.

50. D. A1AT deficiency has several genotypes and can cause cirrhosis as well as bronchiectasis and early emphysema, but does not cause infertility, nor does CVID. CF is the most common congenital cause but the history of ear infections suggests otitis media which is common in PCD. Male infertility in CF due to congenital bilateral absence of vas deferens, in PCD secondary to poor sperm motility. Postinfectious bronchiectasis is a diagnosis of exclusion.

REFERENCES AND ESSENTIAL GUIDELINES

Chapter	Group	Guideline Title	Date
All Chapters	JRCPTB	Specialty Training Curriculum for Respiratory Medicine	2010
Chapter 2 Obstructive lung disease	GINA	Pocket guide for asthma management and prevention	2009
	BTS SIGN	British guideline on the management of asthma	2011
	NICE	Technology appraisal 133: Asthma (uncontrolled) - omalizumab.	2007
	NICE	Clinical guideline 101: Chronic obstructive pulmonary disease	2010
	GOLD	Pocket guide to COPD diagnosis, management and prevention	2009
	NICE	Public health guidance 10: Smoking cessation services	2008
	BTS	BTS statement on pulmonary rehabilitation	2001
Chapter 3 Thoracic oncology and palliative care	UICC International Union Against Cancer	TNM Classification of Malignant Tumours 7th edition	2009
	NICE	Clinical guideline 121: Lung cancer	2011
	BTS Society for Cardiothoracic Surgery	Guidelines on the radical management of patients with lung cancer	2010
	Fleischner Society	Guidelines for management of small pulmonary nodules detected on CT Scans	2005
	GMC	Treatment and care towards the end of life	2010
Chapter 4 Pulmonary infection	BTS	Guidelines for the management of community acquired pneumonia in adults	2009
	BTS British Infection Society Health Protection Agency	Hospital management of adults with severe acute respiratory syndrome	2004
Chapter 5 Tuberculosis and opportunistic mycobacterial disease	NICE	Clinical guideline 117: Tuberculosis	2011
	BTS	BTS recommendations for assessing risk and for managing *Mycobacterium tuberculosis* infection and disease in patients due to start anti-TNFα treatment	2005
	BTS	Guidelines for the prevention and management of Mycobacterium tuberculosis disease in adult patients with chronic kidney disease	2010
	BHIVA	Guidelines for the treatment of TB/HIV co-infection	2010
	BTS	Management of opportunistic mycobacterial infections	1999

Chapter	Group	Guideline Title	Date
Chapter 6 Bronchiectasis	BTS	Guideline for non-CF bronchiectasis	2010
	Royal Brompton Hospital	Clinical guidelines: care of children with cystic fibrosis. 5th edition. www.rbht.nhs.uk/childrencf	2011
Chapter 7 Interstitial lung disease	ATS ERS	International multidisciplinary consensus classification of the idiopathic interstitial pneumonias	2002
	BTS Thoracic Society of Australia and New Zealand Irish Thoracic Society	Interstitial lung disease guideline	2008
Chapter 8 Pulmonary vascular disease	BTS	Guidelines for the management of suspected pulmonary embolism	2003
	ESC	Guidelines on the diagnosis and management of acute pulmonary embolism	2008
	RCOG	Green Top Guideline 37b: The acute management of thromboembolic disease in pregnancy and the puerperium	2007
	BCSH	Guidelines on anticoagulation with warfarin: 4th edition	2011
	National pulmonary hypertension centres of the UK and Ireland	Consensus statement on the management of pulmonary hypertension in clinical practice in the UK and Ireland	2008
	ESC ERS	Guidelines for the diagnosis and treatment of pulmonary hypertension	2009
Chapter 9 Eosinophilic lung disease	—	—	—
Chapter 10 Sleep disorders	SIGN	Guideline 73: Management of obstructive sleep apnoea/hypopnoea syndrome in adults	2003
	NICE	Technology appraisal 139: Continuous positive airway pressure for the treatment of obstructive sleep apnoea/hypopnoea syndrome	2008
	DVLA	At a glance guide to the current medical standards of fitness to drive	2011
Chapter 11 Disorders of the mediastinum and pleura	BTS	BTS Pleural disease guideline	2010
Chapter 12 Occupational and environmental lung disease	BTS	Standards of care for occupational asthma	2008
	BTS	Pleural plaques: information for health professionals	2011
	BTS	Statement on malignant mesothelioma in the United Kingdom	2007
	BTS	Managing passengers with stable respiratory disease planning air travel: British Thoracic Society recommendations	2011
	BTS	British Thoracic Society guidelines on respiratory aspects of fitness for diving	2003
Chapter 13 Lung transplantation	International Society for Heart and Lung Transplantation	International Guidelines for the Selection of Lung Transplant Candidates	2006

Chapter	Group	Guideline Title	Date
Chapter 14 Invasive and non-invasive ventilation	RCP BTS Intensive Care Society	The use of non-invasive ventilation in the management of patients with chronic obstructive pulmonary disease admitted to hospital with acute type II respiratory failure	2008
Chapter 15 Pulmonary function tests	BTS	Spirometry in practice: a practical guide to using spirometry in primary care. 2nd edition	2005
	ATS	Guidelines for the 6-MWT	2002
Chapter 16 Respiratory scoring systems and statistics	—	—	—

INDEX